610.73

KT-500-046

Y & INFORMATION SERVICE
DISTRICT HOSPITAL

Core Skills for Nurse Practitioners

Core Skills for Nurse Practitioners

A Handbook for Nurse Practitioners

Diane Palmer BSc(Hons), RN, PGCE
University of Hull

and

Surrinder Kaur BSc(Hons), RN, RM, CertEd, MTD
Commission for Health Improvement

SERIES EDITORS
Graeme Duthie MD, FRCS(Ed), FRCS
and
Diane Palmer BSc(Hons), RN, PCGE

W
WHURR PUBLISHERS
LONDON AND PHILADELPHIA

© 2003 Whurr Publishers
First published 2003 by
Whurr Publishers Ltd
19b Compton Terrace, London N1 2UN, England and
325 Chestnut Street, Philadelphia PA 19106, USA

All rights reserved. No part of this publication may be
reproduced, stored in a retrieval system, or transmitted in any
form or by any means, electronic, mechanical, photocopying or
otherwise, without the prior permission of Whurr Publishers
Limited.

This publication is sold subject to the conditions that it shall not,
by way of trade or otherwise, be lent, resold, hired out, or
otherwise circulated without the publisher's prior consent in any
form of binding or cover other than that in which it is published
and without a similiar condition including this condition being
imposed upon any subsequent purchaser.

British Library Cataloguing in Publication Data
A catalogue record for this book is available from the British
Library.

ISBN: 1 86156 275 6

Typeset by HWA Text and Data Management, Tunbridge Wells
Printed and bound in the UK by Athenaeum Press Limited, Gateshead, Tyne & Wear

Contents

Contributors

Aldine Alsop MPhil, BA, Dip COT SROT, *Principal Lecturer and Discipline Leader, Occupational Therapy Manager, South Yorkshire Workforce Development Confederation*

Sue Baker RN, M*acmillan CNS Breast Care Nurse, Scarborough Hospital*

Lynda Buckingham MBA, BSc, RGN, RNT, *Director, Unit of Health Services Management, Hull Business School*

Julie Dickinson MEd, DMS, FETC, PGDipHE, CertHE, CertDT, *Lecturer, University of Hull*

Julie D'Silva RGN, FETC, *Consultant Nurse in Gastroenterology, Rotherham Hospital*

Maggie Griffiths RN, BS(Hons), MSOCSci, *Griffiths Bruce Associates*

Tracey Heath RGN, MSc, BSc (Hons),*Lecturer/Senior Nurse Evidence-Based Practice, University of Hull/Northern Lincolnshire and Goole NHS Trust*

Pauline Hutson BA(Hons), RGN, Dip PSN, *Patient Services Manager/Nurse Specialist, Barnsley District General NHS Trust*

Kate Jagger BEd, PG Dip Management, RNT, RCNT, RGN, *Consultant in Professional Development*

Stella Jones-Devitt BA(Hons), MEd, MSc, *Lecturer, University of Hull*

Surrinder Kaur BA(Hons), RN, RM, Cert Ed, MTD, *Review Manager, Commission for Health Improvement*

James M. Mercer MA, BSc(Hons), DipN(Lond), Cert Ed, RGN, *Tutor in Nursing Studies, University of Hull*

Diane Palmer BSc(Hons), RN, PGCE, *Lecturer in Nursing, University of Hull*

Marian Pearson RGN, Dip Ed Dev, *Divisional Nurse, Leeds Teaching Hospitals NHS Trust*

Angela Turner RN, RSCN, FETC, PG Dip (Quality Assurance and Social Care), *Formerly Executive Nurse Director, Sherwood Forest Hospital Trust*

Series Foreword

This series represents a significant addition to the nursing literature. The editors are respected experts and they have assembled a team of authors with the necessary experience and reputation to ensure the authority of each volume. From the stable of the prestigious specialist nurse endoscopy course at the University of Hull and based in the Hull and East Yorkshire Hospitals NHS Trust, this series will ensure that excellence will not be the preserve of these institutions.

Gastroenterology is an important field where nurses can develop and practise as specialist and advanced practitioners. The field extends from the inexplicable, such as irritable bowel syndrome, through the aetiological puzzle of inflammatory bowel disease, to life-threatening malignancies. Irritable bowel syndrome and inflammatory bowel disease both involve significant psychological morbidity and treatment in these areas is ripe for the development of nursing interventions such as counselling and behavioural therapies. Definitive diagnosis of inflammatory disorders and malignancies requires endoscopy, and this is an area where nursing makes a significant contribution through independent practice. Endoscopy is an invasive procedure which raises significant anxiety in patients and one where nurses are able to combine their psychosocial and technical skills. As such, nurses require well developed psychosocial skills – which are integral to nursing practice – and a deep knowledge of the anatomy and physiology of the gastrointestinal tract. The series will ensure that all nurses, particularly those who wish to practise in the field of gastroenterology, will have a sound foundation.

Roger Watson BSc, PhD, RGN, CBiol, FIBiol, ILTM, FRSA
Professor of Nursing, University of Hull

Preface

In assembling this book, we have aimed to establish a text which senior nurses can utilise to support their clinical knowledge and responsibilities.

As two people heavily involved in the nurse endoscopy programmes at Hull University and Castle Hill Hospital, we felt it important that advanced practitioners were comfortable with some core issues as they developed what in many cases are new, revolutionary roles. In Chapter 1, some of the topics which emerged in determining this new role for nurses are discussed. From those discussions evolved a 'core curriculum' for advanced practitioners and senior clinical nurses. The remaining chapters in this book are based on what we now recognise as the core curriculum subjects.

As we approached people to work with us on this book, contributors were encouraged to focus on the needs of clinical nurses who were possibly fairly new to a nurse specialist role. Some of the contributors are from gastroenterology nursing backgrounds and we have asked them to relate examples to their familiar clinical areas. However all of the chapters provide advice which has relevance in any area of nursing.

In addition to clinical knowledge, every senior clinical nurse should be comfortable with the issues addressed in this book. The authors have been specifically selected to provide applied knowledge, which has been tested and utilised in acute hospital environments. We therefore felt able to permit the contributors a broad approach in their chapter preparation, to allow sharing from experience. As editors we are pleased with the individual distinctive styles of each chapter, which we have tried not to tamper with too much, as we believe that content is more relevant than formation.

Some but not all of the chapters have study exercises for the reader to consider. Once again, we have allowed the contributors to determine the appropriateness of such a style to their chapter.

Whilst the initial focus for this book was on the 'novice' nurse specialist, we feel that the result is a core text, which will be of use to many advanced practitioners and nurse specialists, novice and expert alike. In the busy day of the advanced/senior clinical nurse it can be difficult to obtain advice about issues such as lifelong learning, evidence-based care or clinical governance, and this book provides information on such topics.

Developing new roles and ways of working can be pioneering, which in turn brings excitement, loneliness and anxiety, as traditional boundaries are pushed back. This book aims to provide the reader with a number of frameworks, which may assist in developing practice. These will range from developing business cases for new roles, to establishing practice development frameworks. New ways of working require leadership skills and the ability to manage risks whilst initiating changes in a planned, systematic manner. This book provides the reader with a number of perspectives to consider when planning their journey.

Diane Palmer and Surrinder Kaur
August 2002

CHAPTER 1

Practice development

SURRINDER KAUR

Introduction

In 1995, East Yorkshire NHS Trust developed two courses – namely, the English National Board (ENB) Flexible Sigmoidoscopy Course for Nurse Practitioners and the ENB Upper Gastro-Intestinal Course for Nurse Practitioners. They were the first of their kind in the UK at the time. Frost (1998) reports that the ENB received mixed reactions to the latter course. The correspondence to the ENB expressed 'outrage' and 'concern that nursing would be greatly harmed by moving into areas of medical practice'. The debate focused around the essence of nursing being compromised by nurses taking on medical duties. Others congratulated the ENB for enabling 'nurses to develop new and complex skills, to take new responsibilities and develop practice in different and innovative ways' (Frost, 1998).

The aims of this chapter are to:

- explore the drivers for creating the environment for changing practice
- describe the framework to develop practice
- debate whether the level of practice is specialized or advanced.

It also explores the practice development framework (PDF) in which these nurse practitioner posts were cultivated and the use of the framework in the course. The criteria for the PDF were adapted from the University of Leeds Nursing and Practice Development Accreditation Scheme (1992). As an accreditation panel member I had first-hand knowledge that the criteria worked. I had also adapted the criteria to develop practice across the Trust without needing to formally develop Nursing Development Units. The PDF is a way of planning how innovative practice can be systematically created in a defined clinical area for all nurses who wish to

1

move practice forward. The criteria that make up the PDF form the themes of this book, which the authors explore in further detail.

The notions of specialist practice and advanced practice require exploration and are discussed later in this chapter. At the time the new roles were developed, it was difficult to decide what the nurses should be called. The title 'nurse practitioner' was chosen to depict a different role from the traditional roles of nurses working in endoscopy, general surgical wards and clinical nurse specialist roles. At the same time, it was recognized that the roles did not fall neatly into the advanced/consultant role, and it is acknowledged that the use of a variety of terms to depict levels of practice has generated confusion. Before proceeding further, it is necessary to identify the context in which the new roles developed and the management of the change by the employing organization.

The context for change

The development of the nurse practitioner roles occurred in a very short time frame. The factors that allowed this can be defined as the drivers for change. *The Scope of Professional Practice* (UKCC, 1992) was the vehicle that enabled nurses to expand their practice. The formation of an Academic Surgical Unit within the Trust enabled the development of multiprofessional learning and working as well as research to be undertaken within the context of gastroenterology. In the case of the nurses undertaking flexible sigmoidoscopy examinations, the driver was the Academic Surgical Unit's position as a site involved in a national research project, which involved screening for colorectal cancer. It was recognized that there would not be enough medical staff to undertake this and therefore new roles for nurses were needed. At the same time, it was recognized that the development of a 'one-stop' colorectal clinic would benefit patients by streamlining investigations, diagnosis and consultation into a single visit. The care of the patient could be enhanced by a nurse undertaking the counselling and screening, and by following up patients requiring care in the surgical wards. The new role would also involve genetic counselling of families. This type of role was developed in the US and has been very successful.

It is important to think about the potential resistance to change (see Table 1.1) and to plan how it can be minimized or eliminated when developing new roles, although in this instance the resistance to change was minimal.

There are a number of ways in which resistance to the development of new roles can be minimized. First, by having clarity about the need for the

Table 1.1 Drivers and resistance

Drivers for change	Resistance to change
• UKCC Scope of Professional Practice • New Deal – junior doctors' hours (NHS Management Executive, 1991) • Screening for Colorectal Cancer Research Project • Development of 'one-stop clinics' to ensure delivery of services were streamlined to patients • National and local desire to develop new roles to deliver care in flexible ways, e.g. clinical governance, Health Improvement Programmes, National Service Frameworks • General public demanding a more efficient and effective delivery of service • Support from the trust board • Good nursing leadership • Good leadership from the surgical academic unit to promote multiprofessional learning and working • Good partnership working with the higher educational institution • Support from the English National Board	• Perceived erosion of nursing skills at the expense of undertaking medical tasks • Concern that the service would be task orientated • Perceived effects on medical training and junior doctors' experience

role and the benefits to the patient. To do this, it is important to present a case for the role and to discuss it with the professionals on whom it will have an impact, as well as presenting it to the Trust's Executive Management Board and Trust Board. Table 1.2 lists the issues that need to be considered to prepare a case effectively.

By spending time formulating a case, the potential questions that may arise can be thought about and answers prepared. The case can then be adapted for different audiences. It is also important to draw up a list of people who need to be influenced to support your case, with a plan of how you will approach this. Identify who will be your key allies in enabling the change to be supported and implemented. Next consider what resistance there may be and why, and prepare how you will minimize it. When developing the job description, obtain comments from a variety of people who will be affected by the role, and obtain views on the induction, training and development of the person for the new role.

Table 1.2 Preparation for 'Case of need' presentation

- A literature review relating to the proposed change
- Visits to or communications with other organizations that have introduced similar changes
- Presentation of a case for the new role in the form of a report in which you:
    - write an executive summary that simply outlines the need for the change, the options considered and the final option chosen, concluding with the key recommendations to implement the option
    - write an introduction stating the purpose of the report and highlighting the issues or problems that the service is facing, which would benefit from the new role and approach to care
    - identify clearly the aims and objectives of your case
    - link to national policy initiatives e.g. Health Needs Assessment, Health Improvement Programmes, National Service Frameworks
    - present concisely and clearly the facts currently relating to the service. The facts could relate to patient charter standards that are being compromised, patient satisfaction, complaints, the views of staff, the level of service given versus the level of service demanded by patients and general practitioners, the financial costs, loss of opportunity costs
    - write about the advantages and disadvantages of at least three options that could be considered to improve the situation. This can include a 'do nothing' option
    - identify the best option. If this is about developing a new role or a new change, give brief evidence from the literature to support it
- write a conclusion from which recommendations for the future can be made. Write the recommendations in the form of an action plan, with clear timescales attached

The climate has now changed nationally with the publication of *Making a Difference* (DoH, 1999a) and *Saving Lives: our healthier nation* (DoH, 1999b), and the introduction of nurse consultant posts (DoH, 1999c). *The NHS Plan* (DoH, 2000) positively encourages new roles and new ways of working. Nevertheless, the introduction of a new role requires careful planning and management.

The management of change

When considering the development of a new role that expands the boundaries of traditional nursing practice, the organization needs to consider how the role will be supported and developed. The risk management issues need to be identified and a plan to minimize the risks developed. For the Trust to undertake vicarious liability on behalf of the employee, the role needs to be approved by the Trust Management Board.

Risk can be minimized through the development of guidelines and protocols that the new role can operate within. Education and professional support can reduce clinical risks further; these issues can be addressed through the Trust Clinical Governance Strategy and Risk Management Strategy. In the case of nurses expanding their practice to undertake upper and lower endoscopies, it was decided to develop courses that were professionally approved by the ENB to ensure the public were exposed to practitioners who were safe to undertake the new roles. The new roles also developed the scope of nursing practice and ensured a holistic model of care was delivered to patients.

The courses were developed in partnership with the local higher education institution and the ENB.

The PDF formed a key theme within the courses, which would enable practitioners to continue to develop their practice during and after completion of the course. Each criterion was discussed and included in the overall theme of the course. As part of the final assessment, the course participants were asked to produce a practice development plan based on the criteria and guidelines listed below. The plans were presented to all the course participants and their managers, and were then discussed.

Practice development business plan

A business plan is a working tool that enables the practitioner to clearly identify the goals to be achieved in the service. The plan gives direction and can be revised in the light of new unexpected developments. The business plan should be developed jointly with other professionals involved in the delivery of the gastroenterology service. In this way there is ownership and a common understanding of what is to be achieved. By leading on the formulation of a business plan for the development of clinical practice in the gastroenterology service, the course participants gained the co-operation of others, and enabled staff groups to understand the new role and its contribution to the delivery of care. It was also an opportunity to begin to exercise leadership and start to think and plan strategically.

The guidelines given to participants stated that the following attributes should be contained in a business plan:

- the vision of what the service will aim to achieve, in a few sentences
- the clinical areas involved in the business plan
- the leadership role of the nurse practitioner and the model of leadership to be developed in the clinical area
- identification of the multiprofessional team opting into the change by being involved in achieving the objectives of the business plan
- the philosophy of the team in providing a framework of patient care

- the broad aims of the service
- a table setting out the detailed objectives and their implementation (Table 1.3).

Table 1.3 Objective setting

Objective	Key actions to achieve the objective	Success criteria, i.e. what will have been achieved if the objective has been successful	Who will lead on ensuring it will be achieved, who will be involved in helping	The timescale in which the objective will be achieved	Resources required

- the business plan should aim to achieve the objectives within the resources available. There is no logic in devising objectives that are practically unattainable because resources are limited in the form of finance, time or people
- the way in which the objectives will be monitored and reviewed will be identified in the plan
- the plan will identify how the learning from the achievements will be shared within the organization and outside it
- individual personal development plans will need to be in place as part of the practice development framework.

A business plan will enable identification of key stakeholders, which in turn will enable partnership working to develop between different professionals, departments and agencies. The business plan objectives will also help identification of personal objectives for individual performance review. The fact that others will be contributing to the achievement of the objectives will mean that the same applies to them too. This effectively means that the scene is set for all to achieve common ends in a co-operative way. The business plan should link in to the overall organization. It should be informed by the trust business plan as well as any divisional/directorate business plans. This is summarized in Figure 1.1.

Facilitating the development of a practice development business plan

Course participants used a variety of tools to assess what was required to develop a business plan. These included the items shown in Figure 1.2.

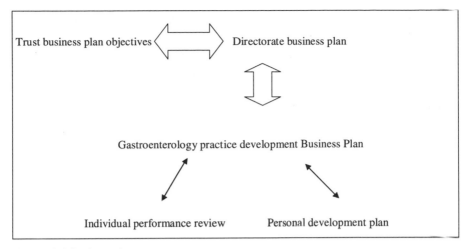

Figure 1.1 Business plans.

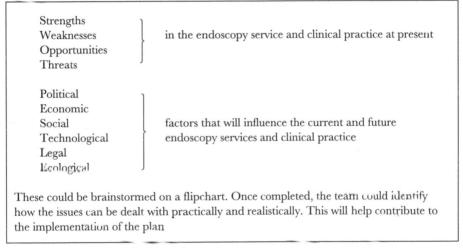

Figure 1.2 Developing a business plan.

The next stage is to develop a vision of what the service and clinical practice will look like in order that patients can readily access the service and receive high-quality care in a timely manner from the appropriate member of staff. This took the form of stakeholders articulating in a short statement what the purpose and aims of the service were and how they were to be achieved. For the nurse practitioner, creating a picture of what the new role would ideally be like and making plans to take steps towards that picture is a positive commitment to that role. It provides an opportunity to think about things differently and to do things differently within the service and care delivery provision.

Having developed a vision, it is important to identify a framework of patient care delivery. This requires articulation of the practitioner's values and beliefs. Course participants analysed a range of theoretical nursing models and transcultural models. They then chose a model or developed an eclectic model in which to frame their care delivery and support patient care documentation development.

By developing a practice development plan the course participants were able to identify a range of initiatives that required development, each set out in priority order. For example:

- setting up nurse-led endoscopy clinics
- developing clinical protocols, guidelines, standards
- development of health promotion activities
- development of patient information and decision-making tools
- development of endoscopy assistant roles
- stating communication and referral processes
- setting up clinical supervision models for themselves
- identifying systems for auditing of practice
- devising documentation to support practice and share multi-professionally.

Leadership

There is a difference between managing and leading. Managerial skills are called for in situations of stability in which goals, tasks, procedures, people and resources are well defined and understood. The manager acts to achieve the goals in the most effective way. Recent health service documents (DoH, 1998, 2000) all stress the importance of leadership to achieving the objectives of the NHS.

Marquis and Huston (2000, p4) list quite distinct differences between managers and leaders, supported by Conger and Kanungo (1998, p9), and these are summarized in Table 1.4.

While many of the course participants were managers of endoscopy services, there was recognition that the development of their role as nurse practitioners would mean letting go of their managerial roles at some stage and concentrating entirely on their new role. They therefore needed to consider the transition from manager to leader, and also to identify how they could develop a shared leadership model with their counterparts in the service to bring about maximum benefit.

Course sessions identified the differences between transactional models of leadership and transformational models of leadership. Participants

Table 1.4 Differences between managers and leaders

Managers	Leaders
• Have assigned managerial positions	• Use their expert or personal power
• Their position has delegated authority and power	• Have a wider variety of roles than do managers
• In order to achieve organizational goals they utilize resources of people, money, time	• Focus on group process, interpersonal skills, gathering information and empowering others
• Have more formal responsibility and accountability for control, allocation and resource management than leaders	• Formulate longer-term strategic objectives
• Direct willing and unwilling subordinates to maintain standards and on-the-job behaviour	• Influence and innovate for the entire service/organization
• Rely on control strategies to get things done, and are able to use sanctions and rewards as formal part of their authority	• Challenge the status quo
	• Use transformational influence to change values, attitudes and behaviour

considered their leadership skills and how they could develop them further. Sashkin and Rosenbach (1993) identified transactional leadership as being about leaders and followers perceiving each other as potentially instrumental in fulfilling each other's needs. Essentially, the leader motivates by appealing to the self-interest of individuals using rewards and sanctions (Bass and Stodgill, 1990). The other end of the continuum, however, relates to transformational leadership, which is about enabling followers to become leaders. Transformational leadership, according to Bass and Stodgill (1990), relates to the leader arousing trust and faith in their abilities through their personality and charisma. The leader is able to intellectually stimulate others in raising the awareness of problems and getting a new perspective on the issue. The leader provides support and encouragement to others and inspires them by communicating a vision to fulfil higher and higher expectations. When working in organizations, nurse practitioners need to consider how they will develop partnerships to bring about changes in practice. Leadership behaviour involves networking and partnership building. To do this, the nurse practitioner will need to build relationships with and between people to share a common purpose and way of working with one another.

Leadership is important for the delivery of good-quality patient care. By influencing the adoption of evidence-based guidelines, protocols and practice, the nurse practitioner can change and develop practice. Leadership can impact on the organization because many practice development initiatives can be shared and adapted in different parts of the organization. The practice development plan will have a dissemination strategy that will help the nurse practitioner and colleagues to share the lessons learnt through publications, presentations, conference papers and poster presentations. The many networks and formal groups within an organization can play a role in dissemination and help to fast-track learning.

Collaboration with higher education

Partnership working with universities is essential in the development of new roles and practices. The involvement of a university in developing and supporting a practice development plan can be invaluable. A lecturer working in close collaboration can act as a critical friend as well as being called on to act as a facilitator, adviser and researcher as necessary. The university is not simply a resource which provides workshops or courses for participants, but can play a critical role in providing consultancy.

Table 1.5 shows areas in which Trusts and higher education institutions may collaborate.

Table 1.5 NHS Trust and higher education collaboration

- Literature searches
- Training needs analysis and the development of new courses
- Facilitation of team building, visioning, business planning
- Project management
- Development of a patient care framework
- Introducing evidence-based practice
- Designing research and audit tools to use in practice
- Developing and providing clinical supervision, mentorship
- Providing support to disseminate information, e.g. writing and presentation skills

So far it can be seen that for the individual and the service to be successful, there needs to be a clear case for developing new roles and a framework in which practice can develop. It is important to have a steering group in place to oversee this, and this should comprise key individuals who can effect organizational change, e.g. director of nursing, consultant, educationalist, non-executive director as well as senior mangers and patient representatives. The role of a steering group is to assist in providing strategic guidance, advise and help in the implementation of plans.

Having established a case for a new role and a practice development business plan, the nurse has the framework in place to specialize further, advance practice or to move towards a nurse consultant role.

Many authors have written about the distinctions and confusion surrounding nursing roles and practice. This chapter is not intended to develop the academic arguments relating to this matter, but to share the type of exercise used to facilitate the discussion with course participants. They were asked to consider which of the criteria identified in the literature they thought applied to their practice and new roles, and why. This involved taking criteria or lists developed by various authors in the literature and asking the following questions.

- How do you define your role and practice in relation to the literature on specialist roles and advancing practice?
- What leads you to this conclusion?
- How do you think you can develop your role or practice to meet the criteria identified?
- How would you explain the similarities and differences between your role and the role of the specialists, advanced nurse practitioners and emerging consultant nurses in your organization?

Table 1.6 on page 12 shows the types of list used to generate the debate.

In conclusion, it must be recognized that in the development of a new role, initially there may be no formal route of preparation or qualifications because of the very nature of the innovative development. Essentially the nurse will have to 'grow' into the role and develop the framework of preparation for others to follow. The nurse can do this by having a personal and practice development plan to facilitate a systematic approach.

Table 1.6 Similarities and differences between roles

Criteria for clinical nurse specialist (CNS) role (Castledine, 1998)	Characteristics of advanced practice (Read, 1998)
• Involvement in patient care • Educated to degree-level, possible Masters degree • Involved in research • Involved in educational programmes for the healthcare team and patients • Co-ordinates care with other healthcare professionals or leads the organization of the patients' total healthcare • Able to act in a consultancy capacity • Concerned with the dissemination of practice in publications and conferences • Acts as a liaison between hospital and community • Has freedom and flexibility in the role	• Expands/adjusts the boundaries of practice • Pioneering • Sophisticated use of clinical knowledge and skill • Systematic assessment of patients leading to healthcare intervention • Independent clinical decision-making • Demonstration of high levels of accountability, autonomy, risk taking • Grounded in nursing theory and practice when making decisions • Educational qualifications beyond registration (Based on Sparacino and Durand, 1986)
Nurse consultants (DoH, 1999c)	**Extended role nurse (Roberts-Davis, 1998)**
• 50 per cent of time spent working directly with patients and clients or communities • Experienced experts in their field • Exercise a high degree of personal professional autonomy and make critical judgements based on advanced knowledge • Make decisions where precedents do not exist • Advise where standard protocols do not exist • Prescribing rights where legislation permits • Provide professional leadership • Contribute to longer-term strategic planning • Contribute to the education of healthcare professionals • Develop professional practice • Will have a track record of scholarship and application of research in practice • Have a portfolio of career-long learning up to or beyond Masters degree level	• 70–80 per cent of time is spent in clinical practice • Educated to Masters level • Performs comprehensive patient assessments based on completing medical and physical examinations to arrive at a nursing and medical diagnosis • Identifies and orders and interprets specific diagnostic tests and procedures • Prescribes specific medication and therapeutic interventions • Independently performs selected invasive or non-invasive medical procedures • Authorizes and co-ordinates admission, discharge and medical follow-up • Has advanced knowledge of educational theory to develop innovative educational programmes for patients and healthcare professionals • Provides expert knowledge to policy and procedure development • Provides leadership by advancing nursing knowledge through research-related activities

References

Bass BM, Stodgill R (1990) Handbook of Leadership Theory, Research and Managerial Applications, 3rd edn. New York: Free Press.

Castledine G (1998) Clinical nurse specialists in the UK; 1980s to the present day. In: Advanced and Specialist Practice. Oxford: Blackwell Science.

Conger JA, Kanungo RN (1998) Leadership in Charismatic Organisations. California: Sage Publications.

Department of Health (1998) A First Class Service: quality in the new NHS. London: Stationery Office.

Department of Health (1999a) Making a Difference: strengthening the nursing, midwifery and health visiting contribution to health care. London: The Stationery Office.

Department of Health (1999b) Saving Lives: our healthier nation. London: The Stationery Office.

Department of Health (1999c) Nurse, Midwife and Health Visitor Consultants: establishing posts and making appointments. Health Service Circular, HSC 1999/217. London: Department of Health.

Department of Health (2000) The NHS Plan: a plan for investment. A plan for reform. London: The Stationery Office.

Frost S (1998) Perspectives on advanced practice: an educationalist's view. In: Rolfe G, Fulbrook P, Advanced Nursing Practice. Oxford: Butterworth Heinemann.

Marquis BL, Huston CJ (2000) Leadership Roles and Management Functions in Nursing, 3rd edn. Philadelphia, Pa: Lippincott Williams and Wilkins.

NHS Management Executive (1991) Junior Doctors, The New Deal. Working arrangements for hospital doctors and dentists in training. London: Department of Health.

Read SM (1998) Exploring new roles for nurses in the acute sector. Professional Nurse 14(2), 90–94.

Roberts-Davis M (1998) Advanced nursing practice: lessons from the province of Ontario, Canada. In: Rolfe G, Fulbrook P, Advanced and Specialist Practice. Oxford: Blackwell Science.

Sashkin M, Rosenbach WE (1993) A new leadership paradigm. In: Rosenbach WE, Taylor RL, Contemporary Issues in Leadership, 3rd edn. Boulder, Colo: Westview Press.

Sparacino P, Durand B (1986) Specialism in advanced practice. Editorial. Momentum 4(2), 2–3.

UKCC (1992) Scope of Professional Practice. London: United Kingdom Central Council for Nursing, Midwifery and Health Visiting.

University of Leeds (1992) Centre for the Development of Nursing, Policy and Practice, Development Accreditation Scheme. http://www.leeds.ac.uk/healthcare/

CHAPTER 2

Leadership

ANGELA TURNER

Introduction

In this chapter the issue of leadership in nursing at the clinical interface is explored with the intention of giving the reader an insight into the complexities of leadership within the nursing profession. Further reading on the subject of leadership is encouraged and is easily referenced manually or electronically in the many journals and libraries nationally and internationally.

In recent times the notion of leadership within the nursing profession has been the subject of intense debate. It probably would be true to say that clinical nurses who manage wards and departments, clinics and patient caseloads do not necessarily see themselves as 'leaders' in the true sense of the word, other than that which their title implies. The senior nurse on the team may have the title ward leader or team leader, but are they empowered to lead?

This is one of the most challenging and potentially rewarding times to be involved in the nursing profession. Never before has leadership been a more important concept to the practice and the profession of nursing. Appropriate leader behaviour is dependent on conditions found in the situation and those affected by the situation.

The importance of experience in the development of leaders has been well described in the literature and it is recognized that successful leaders provide evidence for the need of both knowledge and reasoning. This is important in times of organizational change such as is taking place in the current healthcare system.

It is no longer acceptable to promote individuals just because they are willing to do the job and face the challenges; they must be able to demonstrate potential if not actual leadership or management qualities when applying for these crucial posts. The appointment of poor leaders to senior positions can be costly to an organization if their leadership style is not conducive or sensitive to those they represent or manage.

It is perhaps significant that it is only in recent times that nurses have viewed their senior colleagues as leaders, especially those who are in the public domain or those in the most senior posts in the UK. More recently the trend has been to identify leaders at every level, whether they manage wards (ward leaders) or health centres or larger groups of nurses. In fact, the title 'ward leader' is linked with leadership, but do ward leaders lead? Interestingly, the leadership style of ward leaders has been the focal point for debate for a long time and yet rarely do we find wards and departments managed and led in the same way.

Anecdotally we know that wards, departments and clinics are run by nurses who have very similar management experience and clinical skills, but the views of their staff, colleagues and patients will define their experience of leadership traits very differently. An illustration of how nurses feel about promotion to ward leader status is summed up as follows: 'It was clear that despite being a good clinical nurse I was ill-prepared for my role as a ward leader.'

In order to be successful, ward leaders or ward managers (as their titles imply) must be able to lead and manage. Their roles as staff nurses do not adequately prepare them for this task and frequently we hear of the frustrations and difficulties they face in the everyday clinical environment.

Many of us learned to be clinical leaders by trial and error, by selecting our own role models and by developing our own peer support. Yet the nature of the role and the complexity of today's health service require that specific training and education are fundamental if ward leaders are to meet the demands made on them.

In recognition of the growing complexities of caring for patients in an increasingly technical environment and the creation of subspecialisms within clinical care, the notion of the clinical nurse specialist (CNS) began to emerge. The development of the CNS role in the 1980s and 1990s was preceded in the mid 1960s by the role of the nursing officer. The nursing officer role was introduced as an opportunity for ward sisters to extend their clinical function. Arguably a CNS type of role was envisaged but did not emerge.

The lack of clear role definition for the nursing officers meant that the roles took a managerial path rather than a clinical expansion of role as was initially envisaged. Lack of education and training opportunities also compounded an increasingly unhappy situation. Ward sisters whose skill and abilities within clinical teams had been described as a major strength had their status suddenly diminished and were now treated with derision and taunts with jibes such as clip board carriers, this unfortunate state of affairs leading eventually to the demise of the nursing officer role.

The introduction by the UKCC of the *Scope of Professional Practice* offered nurses more flexibility and the opportunity to enhance and expand their role in response to various drivers for change (Todd, 1997). The UKCC defined specialist nurses as nurses who 'exercise higher levels of judgement, discretion and decision making in clinical care. They will be able to monitor and improve standards of care through supervision of practice, clinical audit, the provision of skilled professional leadership and the development of practice through research, teaching and support of professional colleagues' (UKCC, 1992).

Since the mid-1990s, the CNS has emerged as a significant and increasingly important member of the multidisciplinary team. Interestingly, their roles have had a similar pattern of development to that described earlier for the nursing officers' role. It is apparent that some nurse specialists have developed their roles both as a team player and individual beyond the parameters of the original guidance, and yet evidence suggests that there are those clinical nurse specialists who have not developed their roles at all. It is also apparent that despite clinical nurse specialists with innovative and creative roles and extended or specialist skills, many CNSs still perceive themselves to be lacking leadership skills.

To establish a baseline of the extent to which CNSs believe themselves to be leaders in the clinical setting, a small study involving the development of a short questionnaire was designed and distributed to the CNSs within one single acute trust.

A total of 19 CNSs were surveyed and each of the respondents completed a short six-part questionnaire based on their roles within their speciality. They were asked the following :

1 To explain their role as a leader
2 To indicate in what circumstances they 'led'
3 To determine the qualities they possessed as a leader
4 If others (line managers, subordinates, peers, professional colleagues) regarded them as leaders, how this was demonstrated
5 What, if any, training they had received for their roles as leaders
6 What skills they had subsequently developed in their roles as leaders.

In addition, the respondents were also asked to indicate how long they had been in post.

Responses

The shortest length of time in post was two months, the longest 14 years. Between them, they had 87 years and five months' experience as clinical nurse specialists.

Question 1. Explanation of their role as a 'leader'

All the clinical nurse specialists responded to this question and, as expected, the responses varied considerably. Several responded that they delegated tasks, that they shared knowledge with their teams, offered up-to-date knowledge on procedures and were able to cascade information to others. Other respondents broadened their responses to include 'acting as a resource to promote sound evidence-based practice'. Examples include: 'I initiated and maintained the nurse-led preoperative assessment service, which involved a great deal of change within medical and nursing practice'; 'A large part of my role is both role model and evaluator of current practice against national standards and evidence base instigating new practices'.

Question 2. In what circumstances they led

Responses to this were consistent with responses from question 1, and included:

- 'patient advocate, educator, developed multidisciplinary guidelines'
- 'initiating and influencing change'
- 'co-ordinate the multidisciplinary team, strategic communication, motivating and inspiring others to have a vision of what we can do, increasing the confidence of nursing and other multidisciplinary staff'
- 'act as a resource for junior doctors and ward nurses'
- 'developing nursing practice'
- 'teacher, researcher and facilitator'
- 'lecturer and innovator'
- 'advanced nursing assessments in provision of patient information'.

It is at this point in the survey that we are beginning to see trends in their responses and the emergence of some statements about themselves as leaders in their roles as CNSs, but there is also reference to their roles as managers. There is also a trend starting to emerge about the quality of leadership associated with the respondent. It would appear that those

CNSs who are regarded as being at the 'leading edge' and who have national as well as international experience are those who have remained focused on their roles as leaders and not used terminology that could describe management and leadership skills interchangeably. They also seem to have a clear understanding of their roles and are more prone to use words such as vision, innovator and change, or phrases that include evidence-based practice, role model, etc.

The CNSs who responded that they delegated tasks, shared knowledge and were able to cascade information indicate that they 'manage' rather than lead in their specialist area.

This analysis of the questions is by no means definitive but it does raise questions as to the understanding of roles and in what circumstances the clinical nurse specialists lead or manage.

Question 3. What qualities do you possess as a leader?

The responses to this question were interesting and varied, and range from one-word descriptors to examples of how they, as clinical nurse specialists, lead in their field. They included:

- 'The ability to work autonomously, but with the knowledge of organizational and corporate objectives.'
- 'I have the vision, tenacity and an openness to ideas/suggestions, but I rarely deviate from the goal.'
- 'I am often described as dynamic but I feel this is because I am enthusiastic and forward thinking. Personally I feel encouraging ideas, guiding, good communication skills and encouraging others to gain confidence are just as important.'
- '... an ability to stay calm under stressful conditions (I am still perfecting this), able to prioritize workload and to be positive. If there are problems solutions can always be found.'
- '... innovator who has to lead from the front.'
- 'I have established and earned respect from colleagues of all disciplines.'

Other responses included evidence of improved communication, evidence-based practice, a source for information, motivator and assertiveness.

Question 4. Do others regard you as a leader, and how is this demonstrated?

This has four parts. The question is followed by: (a) your immediate line manager, (b) your peers, (c) your subordinates, (d) your professional colleagues.

In relation to part (a), many respondents described being able to work autonomously, having respect for nurse expertise and non-judgemental attitudes. Others explained more fully, and their responses included:

- '... supporting the role and developments or projects to be undertaken.'
- 'We regularly discuss issues of day surgery which impact on inpatient beds/management of waiting lists and formulate possible solutions.'
- 'Possibly views me as a clinical leader (knowledge and expertise) to plan services, but I don't know if she sees me as a leader. She does describe me as dynamic amongst other things!'
- 'Being allowed to get on with my job without interference but having support when it is needed – respect for any ideas and opinions'.

In relation to part (b), 'your peers', responses included:

- 'We learn from one another'.
- 'Contact me for advice.'
- 'See me as an expert in my field.'
- 'Assisted other specialist nurses to set up nurse-led clinics.'
- 'Act as a resource to nurses in other trusts ... by utilising my skills and knowledge.'

In relation to part (c), 'your subordinates', the responses reflected those already outlined in response to parts (a) and (b).

In relation to part (d), 'your professional colleagues', responses included:

- 'Mutual sharing of information and mutual response.'
- '... also asked to provide a certain amount of guidance to junior medical staff.'
- 'Recognition of my contribution.'
- 'Advise surgeons and anaesthetists regarding changes/developments in day surgery practice.'
- 'I am asked for advice on issues such as information about the various schemes. Teaching sessions are arranged to improve understanding.'

- 'An equal in a multidisciplinary setting.'
- 'I am regarded as an expert in my field. I have published articles and presented at national conferences.'
- 'They seek my advice and guidance concerning nursing matters and expect me to know the answers or where to find them.'
- 'Practical skills, e.g. intra-articular injections, patient information, clinical audit.'

From the responses to questions 3 and 4, the qualities the nurse specialists themselves have when compared with the perceptions they have about their roles as perceived by their managers, peers, subordinates and professional colleagues, plot an interesting course of thinking and development in the past few years.

In terms of qualities of leadership, the clinical nurse specialists – and again it is pertinent to those nurse specialists who have been in post several years – view themselves positively and regard themselves to be competent and dynamic within their specialist area. They remain focused but are open to suggestion and aware of the considerable challenges they face.

The relationship that the clinical nurse specialists have with their line manager requires further exploration and is not within the scope of this chapter. However, this brief study poses more questions than it gives answers about relationships between clinical nurse specialists and their line management arrangements and the notion of leadership.

Some of the respondents were very clear and voiced their opinions quite positively. Others – by far the majority – were either unclear as to how to respond to the question or were unsure as to leadership in this context, or both.

As expected, the responses from the clinical nurse specialists in relation to their views about peers and subordinates were very positive, with very clear support for the specialist roles both internally and externally to the Trust in which they work.

In response to part (d) of question 4 there does seem to be significant acceptance of the role of the CNS within the multidisciplinary team. More notably with the medical staff, the truculent attitudes that prevailed in the late 1980s and mid-1990s in being dismissive about the role, expertise and knowledge of clinical nurse specialists have all but disappeared. The acceptance of clinical nurse specialists as credible individuals in their own right is apparent and welcomed, and their leadership qualities are quite definitely acknowledged and accepted.

Queston 5. What training have you received for your role as leader?

Of the 19 clinical nurse specialists surveyed, ten said they had received some training to equip them in their role and nine said they had not.

Of the ten who said they had received training, each of the respondents qualified their answer further. Responses included:

- 'I keep myself updated clinically by reading appropriate journals and attending relevant study days/conferences.'
- 'Informally by learning from other nurses in similar posts…!'
- 'Manager/leader module for BSc(Hons).'
- 'As part of my diploma in nursing I did a leadership module and did some training sessions for leaders, but it was limited and a long time ago.'
- 'Currently undertaking an MBA.'

Some of the comments of the nine participants who said they had not received training are listed below:

- '… skills gained from experience in a leadership position previously, combined with academic study I believe are transferable.'
- 'In my previous role of primary nurse on an acute medical ward, I had already begun developing skills as a leader. These have been developed further whilst in post and "on the job". Having a role model already in post has helped.'
- 'I have studied this during my degree work, but nothing since.'
- 'I have previously undertaken and taught on action-centred leadership courses.'

Question 6. What skills have you developed as a leader?

Responses to this question included:

- 'Improved time management skills … development of autonomous practice.'
- '… knowledge and confidence to take lead in the provision of procedures, guidelines, protocols, etc.'
- 'I have developed planning skills in order to anticipate potential problems and strategies to deal with obstructors.'

- 'To lead more indirectly, no authority to change things but having evidence and earning respect ... takes much longer to change things than you think.'
- 'Managing change creatively.'
- 'I feel that I am always developing skills, particularly the areas which I find naturally quite hard, e.g. keeping focused on the priorities as I would like to do everything at once.'
- 'Getting the best out of people in difficult circumstances.'
- 'Counselling and negotiation skills.'
- 'Delegation skills.'
- 'I am more assertive now. I can offer more support, encouragement and knowledge.'
- 'Confidence in one's ability to lead the profession comes through experience gained in clinical practice, lecturing and by developing interpersonal skills, as well as the ability to communicate effectively.'

The objective of the final questions in this survey was to elicit any training that the clinical nurse specialists may have undergone to equip them with skills as leaders, followed by the skills they had developed in their leadership role.

The responses were predictable in as much as very little formal training had taken place and most skills had been developed 'on the job'. Reading, networking (although not stated explicitly) and attending conferences formed the common denominator of how the clinical nurse specialists acquired their leadership skills.

Reading between the lines of this survey, it can be deduced that leaders of the profession are both made and bred and there is not one single approach to developing such skills. Experience and credibility seem to form the core components of leadership if CNSs are to be accepted as a valuable member of the multidisciplinary team. The evidence suggests that clinical leadership, despite a shaky start, is alive and well and growing.

Benner (1984) describes the development of novice to expert, particularly linked to the inception of the clinical nurse specialist. Her work on this matter has proved to be invaluable to the nursing profession in determining how nurses are developed. The same could be applied to those nurses aspiring to become leaders, recognizing that at some point (and maybe on many occasions) all nurses, midwives and health visitors will find themselves in a leadership position at the clinical interface.

Ward leaders as defined by their role specifications lead teams of nurses and health care assistants; their roles as leaders have emerged as critical to the teams' success. The role of clinical nurse specialist is evolving and is emerging as a pivotal role that is seen as skilled, one that is based on research and evidence-based practice. More crucially, the management of patient care and the acceptance of this role by the clinical teams are firmly embedded within the healthcare setting.

References

Benner P (1984) From Novice to Expert: excellence and power in clinical nursing practice. Menlo Park, Calif: Addison-Wesley.

Todd A (1997) Guidance on the development and implementation of new clinical roles in nursing (unpublished). Trent Region.

UKCC (1992) Scope of Professional Practice. London: United Kingdom Central Council for Nursing, Midwifery and Health Visiting.

CHAPTER 3

Change management

TRACEY HEATH and KATE JAGGER

Change is critical to the growth and success of the profession of nursing. The development of nurse practitioner roles and their impact on care provide testimony to this statement. Change appears to have been a constant feature of healthcare during the past decade. Learning to influence, anticipate and cope with change and to seize the opportunities that it presents are key requirements of any nurse, but particularly those in advanced roles.

This chapter explores change from an individual and an organizational perspective, working from the premiss that in order to effectively promote change and development in others, you must first understand how you deal with and respond to change yourself. The nurse practitioner holds a developing role in a developing service; driving change from within undoubtedly forms part of this role; learning to respond to and deal with external changes effectively will ensure its continued success.

Change can happen accidentally, incrementally and almost imperceptibly, or as a result of a well thought out and deliberate effort. It is the latter or 'planned change' that forms the focus of this chapter.

What is change?

Change has been described as the move from a steady state to one of uncertainty. Whether that uncertainty is perceived positively or negatively depends not only on the change itself, but also the individual's perception of it (Gillies, 1994).

All change, but particularly planned change, represents an opportunity to alter the flow of events. A great deal of change occurs as the result of external triggers. Social and economic factors, political decisions and developments in research and technology can all serve to transform our professional practice. The nurse practitioner needs to keep abreast of advances in the world beyond her department and be able to interpret what any external influences mean for her own role, team or organization. You may like to consider the factors outlined in Table 3.1 and how they affect your working environment.

Change is not simply a matter of responding to external ideas and wishes. The nurse practitioner's role as a leader means that she not only needs to look for better ways of doing things herself but must also encourage and inspire colleagues to do the same. 'Bottom-up' change can be promoted through a formal arrangement such as a practice development or quality group, or just by asking for suggestions. Even simple ideas, if they are seized and followed through, can make a huge difference to the quality of care received by patients.

Table 3.1 Keeping abreast of external change

What are the main forces outside your department that have affected your work within the past few years?	
The following headings may serve as useful triggers when reviewing the forces for change outside your department or organization.	
Political	What government initiatives impact directly or indirectly on your work and that of your department?
Economic	What impact will local or national changes in investment in health have on your practice?
Social	What do demographic changes, changes in lifestyle or public expectations mean for the service you provide?
Technological	What new interventions and technologies are being developed in your field? What new evidence is available to inform your practice?
Legislative	What implications do changes in legislation, for example that related to health and safety, have for your service?
Environmental	What potential impacts do changes in the preferred environment of care or 'environmental-friendly' policies have on your practice?

Adapted from: Morris et al. (2000)

The individual and change

Reactions and resistance

We are all individuals and we see things in different ways; successful change management requires an acceptance of this. Examining your own feelings about change may be a useful first step to understanding the reactions of others. Five categories of people have been identified according to their characteristic attitude and response to change (Rogers, 1983):

- innovators: a small group of experienced, educated and venturesome individuals who are likely to initiate change

- early adopters: respected individuals, calculated in their approach to change and who often act as opinion leaders
- early majority: capable of and happy to change once concrete evidence of its benefit has been accrued
- late majority: sceptical individuals who are generally reluctant to change
- laggards: individuals who are highly reluctant to change and somewhat intransigent.

While this model is not without its critics (you may identify with different groups depending on the nature of the change) it does provide a useful starting point for considering the way in which a new idea may be received by individuals.

Reflection point one: responding to change

Do you identify with one of Rogers' (1983) categories? Do you recognize any of your colleagues in these descriptions? Which category would you prefer to be associated with? Why?

It is doubtful whether anyone reading this text identified herself as a laggard in response to the above exercise. It would be tempting to conclude that laggards are 'trouble' and a 'problem' to be overcome. It almost seems immoral in this day and age to be steadfast in your ways and avoidant of change. However, resistance to change can serve a very useful purpose. It encourages us to be clear about the goals and target of change, to ensure that we can justify our position when questioned and to ensure that the needs of all concerned are carefully considered.

Individuals resist change for a variety of reasons and in a variety of ways. Resistance is not always actively expressed (for example in the form of aggression), but may result in less obvious behaviour such as absenteeism or lethargy. Reflecting on your own experience of change may provide insight into the ways in which disquiet is conveyed.

Altered behaviour may be one way in which the impact of change is expressed, but this in itself says little about the individual's underlying emotional response. Covey (1994) describes personal change as creating a relationship between something you know and something new. Several authors have considered the emotional stages associated with this process (for example, Perlman and Takacs, 1990; Manion, 1998), with those such as Upton and Brooks (1999) suggesting that change may be perceived as a loss and as such invoke a response not dissimilar to grief.

Presumably then some resistance can be expected when those involved perceive that the new regime means significant loss for them, whether this is in the form of established social relationships, status or rewards.

Reflection point two: why people resist change

Reflect for a moment on a time when you have been opposed to change either personally or professionally.

- Why did you resist the introduction of something new or different into your professional or working life?
- Did the change occur anyway?
- Would anything have made the process easier?

In response to reflection point two you may have identified one or more of a variety of issues. Were your values and beliefs threatened? Were your work or personal relationships threatened? Were you worried that you would not cope? Did you feel unprepared for or unclear of what was expected of you? Did you simply not believe that the change held any benefits?

Earlam et al. (2000) identifies four broad categories of resistance:

- cultural: related to the maintenance of values, beliefs and traditions
- social: related to the preservation of existing relationships and teams
- organizational: related to safeguarding time, status or rewards
- psychological: related to fear of the unknown.

Identifying potential sources of resistance when instituting change, or the roots of your own resistance when faced with something new, can be a useful starting point for successful change management. For example, Jones and McDonnell (1993) suggest that resistance will be less if the change accords with established values, those advocating the change understand the feeling and fears of those affected and take steps to relieve them, and if the change is perceived to reduce rather than increase present burdens – in short, if factors contributing to cultural, social, organizational and psychological resistance are addressed.

Resistance to change is not inevitable (a fact that Rogers' (1983) work serves to highlight) but it is not surprising that it does occur. The status quo may appear safe and comfortable, and with any change comes the risk of failure.

As discussed earlier, it may be that the nurse practitioner is subject to, rather than the catalyst for, change. It is important that the nurse practitioner is able to identify sources of support and influence in both situations.

Reflection point three: managing self in times of change

- Make a list of all the means by which you obtain support within your working life.
- What other sources of support exist that you are not currently utilizing?
- Are there any sources of support that you need to create or seek if you are to be effective, not only as an agent of change but as someone able to respond to changing situations?

Support comes in many guises, in the form of mentors, clinical supervisors and professional networks, as well as through less formal, more fluid arrangements. Time spent establishing and developing the sources of support available to both yourself and your colleagues during periods of change is never time wasted.

Even when change is carefully planned and supported, difficulties can still sometimes arise, and while by no means inevitable, no discussion of change would be complete without some reference to conflict and the means by which it can be resolved.

Conflict and its resolution

Conflict, although uncomfortable, is part of everyday life. It is something most people view negatively and would prefer to avoid, yet conflict is not necessarily a bad thing and may lead to positive outcomes (Mullins, 1996).

In the change situation, conflict is manifest in resistance (Huber, 2000) and may have one or more sources. The roots of conflict can lie in:

- perceived differences in values, beliefs and priorities (for example, organizational and individual goals)
- unclear roles and boundaries (resulting in one individual 'encroaching' on another's territory or leaving tasks uncompleted)
- communication and leadership style
- mismatch between the requirements of the role and the individual undertaking it.

This is not an exhaustive list and it may be beneficial to spend time reflecting on your own experience of conflict. It is also worth remembering that the source of conflict may not lie within the existing situation but in unresolved issues from the past. When threatened by a situation, how often does a list of negative incidents arise in our memory to reinforce our stance?

Reflection point four: spend some time reflecting on your own experience of conflict

- What were the causes of the conflict?
- How did you feel?
- How did you deal with those thoughts and feelings?
- How did you resolve the conflict? Did you reach some agreement, or did you bury it inside?
- How did the conflict affect others around you?
- If you did not resolve the conflict, how has it affected your future reaction to a conflict situation?

Identifying the factors underpinning a conflict situation is the first step towards resolving it. Covey (1994, p235) suggests that 'we must seek first to understand – then to be understood'. This is particularly relevant to the resolution of conflict. It may not be the change itself, but its timing or the manner in which it is communicated that is causing problems. The factors contributing to discord will dictate the strategy used to resolve it. However, once the situation has been analysed the nurse practitioner needs her values, beliefs and goals to be understood too. When attempting to bring about change the nurse practitioner may find that she is in collision with the custom or practice of the department or team with which she works. The best way forward may involve compromise, the objective being to create a win–win situation in which all parties feel good about the decision and are committed to the action plan (Covey, 1994).

Conflict resolution

Using the following pointers will help you to create a positive outcome for all concerned.

- Reflect on what is good about the situation. Put the spotlight on what is already working then look at what needs to be changed.
- Create openness and involvement by listening and restating what the other party wants.

- Determine what you want, remembering Covey's (1994, p235) statement, 'seek first to understand then to be understood'.
- Determine what you are willing to do or to give up to get the desired result.
- Establish what the other party is willing to do or to give up, to get what they desire.
- Aim for a win–win solution by establishing mutual goals.
- Find a place for discussion that is considered neutral ground and where you are able to talk about the situation openly without fear of interruption.
- Whenever you are working together adopt a co-operative approach, in which knowledge and expertise are shared.
- Negotiate time out if possible, but remember that conflict needs to be dealt with as it occurs.

Reflection point five: dealing with conflict

Think of a change in practice you have wanted to make recently.

- Did your colleagues share your idea?
- Were there any areas of conflict in relation to the change?
- Why do you think you encountered the conflict?
- Did you deal with the conflict effectively?
- On reflection, which solutions would you keep and what would you do differently in future similar situations?

Most of us will have experienced conflict at some time in our lives and will be aware of its negative effects. By learning to handle discord and disagreement as it arises, the nurse practitioner is in a position to translate this potential problem into a powerful, positive force.

Promoting changes in practice

>...the availability of a committed and skilled nurse who acts as a change agent facilitates the acceptance and management of change.
>
> (NHSE, 1998, p51)

The nurse practitioner is in an ideal position to promote and lead change. The following section represents a distillation of some of the key ideas and principles associated with successful change management, and is intended to promote a systematic approach to this process.

A baffling array of change management theories are in existence, the majority of which were developed within and for industry. However, recent years have witnessed a surge of interest in change management within healthcare, particularly in relation to the development of evidence-based practice (see for example, NHSE, 1998; NHS Centre for Reviews and Dissemination, 1999). For ease of discussion and to serve as an aide-mémoire for the practising nurse the five-point framework outlined in Figure 3.1 will be used to structure the remainder of this chapter.

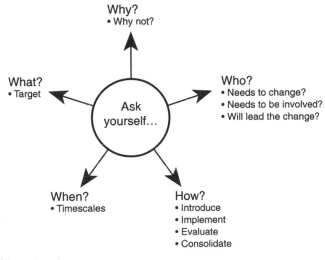

Figure 3.1 Managing change.

What?

Successful instigators of change have a clear vision, they know what they want to achieve and can 'see' it becoming a reality. Being clear about the target of change is the first important principle of successful change management. Generally the focus of change will lie in one or more of three areas: knowledge, attitudes or behaviour (Bernhard and Walsh, 1995).

A change in knowledge level is perhaps the easiest to achieve, usually through the use of various educational strategies. Encouraging someone to overhaul their values and beliefs, or to change an aspect of their behaviour, may be rather more difficult. In practice, attitudes, knowledge and behaviour overlap and influence one another. Many projects, but particularly more complex ones (such as practice development initiatives), require attention to all three areas. Encouraging colleagues to adopt a new practice or expand their role is unlikely to be achieved simply by enhancing their knowledge of the possibilities that exist. Successful change is more likely to result through strategies aimed at modifying their beliefs (about what constitutes the role of the nurse in the endoscopy suite, for example) and assisting them to acquire new skills with which to change practice.

In addition to variations in the focus or target of change, projects also vary in scope. Change may range from an alteration to one aspect of practice to a complete overhaul of the manner in which an entire service is delivered. The person instigating or leading the change needs to be focused, have clear goals and milestones, recognize what is feasible and be realistic about the time it will take.

Who?

Consideration needs to be given at the outset to all those involved in and affected by the change. These individuals are often termed the 'stakeholders'.

Stakeholders are individuals or groups affected by and capable of influencing the change (Swage, 2000). Stakeholders can usefully be considered as those who:

*   hold powers of approval or veto (let it happen)
*   are responsible for action and delivery (make it happen)
*   provide resources (help it happen).

It is not only those who will be directly responsible and undertaking the development that need to be consulted, although these individuals are of course very important to a project's success. Permission may be required, particularly if a development is likely to involve costs, or changes to an individual's role or the service provided by a department.

Changing your own or supporting a change in your nursing colleagues' practice may have implications for the role of other members of the multidisciplinary team. If you or others are relinquishing old or accepting new responsibilities this may involve changes in the role of others and the need to renegotiate boundaries. Furthermore, the potential impact of the change on those individuals who do not work within your immediate environment but another department, such as pharmacy, catering or patient transport, must not be overlooked.

The impact of the change on the patient or client in receipt of the service must also be considered. The introduction of the nurse practitioner role, for example, usually involves patients being asked whether they are happy to be primarily under the care of a nurse rather than the medical consultant. Changes may need to be phased in over a period of time to prevent disruption to those using existing services.

The person leading the change is often termed the change agent (McPhail, 1997). Careful consideration needs to be given with regard to who is the most appropriate person to undertake this role. If the nurse practitioner is acting in this capacity she should be aware of her position in relation to other members of the team and the potential pitfalls and benefits associated with it.

External change agents, that is those from outside the department or organization in question, are sometimes distrusted. If you are in this position, individuals will need to be assured of your motives and believe that you are not only an expert in the field, but are aware of the intricacies of their unique, local situation. Getting local opinion leaders on board (the early adopters identified by Rogers (1983)) is one useful strategy. Who you will need to persuade and how this will be undertaken are important early considerations, particularly if the change is your idea. As an internal change agent, it is important to be objective. Since you are not going to walk away at the end of the change period, consolidating and sustaining the change after the initial period of enthusiasm has faded may seem easier. In either event, if the change is to be successful, it is important that those involved own the change and it is not perceived to be yours. It may be more appropriate for another team member to lead the change and, particularly if the change is 'bottom up' (initiated from within), a leader may emerge during early discussions.

Whether change agents are internal or external, appointed or emerge, McPhail (1997) suggests that to be successful they need to sense the right moment, find supporters for their ideas, have vision, earn trust and respect, demonstrate expert power, and have an effective communication and consultation style. Becoming a change agent is a role not to be undertaken lightly.

Why and why not?

Effective change comes about through choice.

(Taylor, 1999, p164)

The first question we must ask is whether the proposed change is really necessary. Every change has costs associated with it, whether personal or financial. The need to change and the prospect of a better future must far outweigh the costs. Change should be implemented only for good reasons and never simply for change's sake. Change may be gladly welcomed, but it can also be extraordinarily painful and reduce people's capacity to perform (Pattison, 1996).

One popular theory of change, perhaps in part because of its simplicity, is that provided by Kurt Lewin (1951). Lewin views change as the product of two opposing forces: driving forces and restraining forces. In order for change to occur in the desired direction, the drive for change must exceed the forces against change. When driving and restraining forces are equal, a state of equilibrium is maintained and the status quo goes undisturbed. The role of the change agent is therefore to 'unfreeze' the present situation by making a case for the new development. Making a case can usefully be thought of in terms of increasing the driving forces and reducing the restraining forces related to the situation (Figure 3.2).

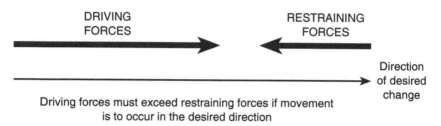

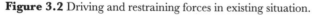

Driving forces must exceed restraining forces if movement is to occur in the desired direction

Figure 3.2 Driving and restraining forces in existing situation.

Many factors influence the process of and decision to change (Table 3.2 provides some general examples), not least of all values and beliefs. Changes in practice need to be consistent with the values and beliefs (usually evident in the departmental philosophy) of those involved. Ethical change involves closely examining these values and beliefs (Collinson, 1999).

People from different occupational groups do not always use terms or see priorities in the same way, and this needs to be taken into account if your proposal for change is to be understood and valued by others. In

Table 3.2 Examples of driving and restraining forces

Driving forces	Restraining forces
Change perceived to be advantageous to patients, professionals and the organization	Lack of time and resources
Change accords with existing values and beliefs	Cost
Change is supported by national or local policy	Lack of support from managers / the organization
Change is supported by up-to-date evidence	Perceived loss of status or rewards
Recognized experts and local opinion leaders support the change	Fear of the unknown
Change appears relatively straightforward	Lack of confidence in ability to adopt new practice
A trial period is possible.	
Benefits will be highly visible	

short, practitioners involved need to see why current practice has to change, believe that the change will work, and feel able to participate if the change is to be embraced.

Reflection point six: before proposing a change in practice or service delivery think carefully

Ask yourself:

- What are the forces driving this change forward?
- Is this change necessary?
- What are the benefits of the change for the patient, the profession, the individual or the organization as a whole?
- What will happen if the change does not take place?
- Which driving forces can be strengthened and how?
- What are the possible sources of resistance to this change?
- Will the change inconvenience or disadvantage anyone, the individual, team or organization?
- Which restraining forces have to be worked with, which can be altered, and how?

How?

> Plan all the way to the end.
>
> (Greene and Elffers, 1999, p105)

No change will occur until the situation has been unfrozen. The importance of planning in the successful management of change should not be underestimated. Planning includes deciding the overall change management strategy to be adopted, in addition to producing a detailed outline of the aims and objectives of the project, the key tasks to be undertaken and resources required.

An example of a simple project plan is provided in Figure 3.3. This format includes the broad aim or purpose of the project, its rationale, specific objectives and an action plan detailing clearly who is to undertake which tasks and by when they should be completed. The need to secure resources (for example, time, money or equipment) should not be overlooked in the planning stage and needs to be included in the written plan, lest it is forgotten.

The SMART formula can be useful in helping to set clear and meaningful objectives (Upton and Brooks, 1999). In short, objectives should be:

- Specific: explicit and unambiguous statements of what is to be achieved.
- Measurable: include criteria for success.
- Achievable: realistic and attainable.

- Relevant: deal with important issues of priority to the organization and the individuals involved.
- Timed: relate to a specified period of time.

Aim
Rationale
Specific objectives

Action Plan

Project co-ordinator_____

Key task	By whom	By when	Review date

Figure 3.3 Example of a simple project plan.

Clarity not only of purpose but of expectations is important if resistance is to be minimized. Each task may involve the efforts of a number of people, but someone needs to be assigned overall responsibility for its completion. When undertaking large or complex projects, a steering group may be required. Steering groups set the overall direction of the project and ensure that it keeps on course, monitoring the progress made against the objectives set. The steering group usually includes key individuals, representative of the groups of stakeholders involved and the project manager or leader.

The analysis of the drivers and restraining factors associated with the proposed change provides useful information regarding the strategies required for successful management. Sources of resistance can be anticipated and, wherever possible, reduced or eliminated, and the drivers for change capitalized upon and reinforced. For example, fear and lack of confidence can be addressed through education and training. Linking it to the departmental or organizational philosophy can reinforce the value of the change.

There is no single ideal strategy for achieving change (Kitson, 1997). Choice of strategy depends on the time available, the relationship between the change agent and those undertaking the change, and the target of change (that is, whether it is a change in behaviour, attitudes, knowledge or a combination of all three that is required).

Three groups of change management strategies have been identified (Chin and Benne, 1985):

- power–coercive
- rational–empirical
- normative–re-educative.

The key features of each strategy are outlined in Table 3.3. The use of more than one strategy is recommended if change is to be long lasting. For example, changing practice may involve an initial period of education and training to facilitate partnership and collaboration later. Reward (in terms of positive feedback) can serve to motivate at all stages. Even in emergency situations, where safety is at risk and a direct approach is vital, later reinforcement with literature and discussion is often advisable.

As discussed earlier, change programmes require sound project management with carefully developed objectives and a realistic timescale if the implementation is to be successful (NHS Centre for Reviews and Dissemination, 1999). If possible, a trial or pilot period should be the first phase of implementation. Not only can this assist in reducing resistance to

Table 3.3 Selecting a strategy for change

Strategy	Techniques	Target	Time	Relationship
Power–coercive	Reward Punishment Telling Command	Behaviour	Fast results designed to achieve compliance in the short term	Change agent has position power and control over sources of reward/punishment
Rational–empirical	Persuasion Selling Informing Explaining Educating	Knowledge	Slower but achieves higher level of certainty	Change agent needs to be viewed as an expert in the field
Normative–re-educative	Participation and delegation	Attitudes and values	Slowest but designed to achieve long-term outcomes	Partnership and collaboration supportive

the new initiative (on the basis that if it does not work during this period it will be abandoned or modified), but it can also serve as a useful test period, during which flaws and problems are addressed before widespread adoption.

A systematic approach and appropriate choice of change management strategy are not the only considerations. Depending on the nature of the change, it may be possible to employ other tools (such as guidelines) to assist in the task of changing practice. The NHSE (1998) provides a useful overview of this area; some of the key approaches are summarized in Figure 3.4. Suffice it to say here that no method is guaranteed to be

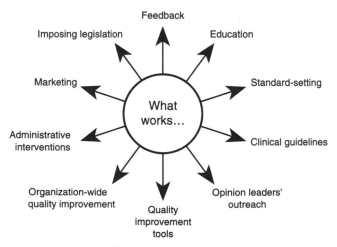

Figure 3.4 Methods of changing clinical practice.

effective, the choice of tool depends on the nature of the development and several approaches in combination are better than one in isolation.

Before embarking on a mission, particularly one to change practice, it is important to ask yourself to what extent you are responsible for the outcome. You can only really change your own practice; you may seek to influence that of your colleagues, but they are the only ones who can really make a difference. While you may be in a position to facilitate the process, they need to own it. When choosing an approach it is helpful to keep this thought in mind.

When?

Preach the need for change but never perform too much at once.

(Greene and Elffers, 1999, p167)

Most people are too ambitious in terms of project size and their estimation of the time it will take to complete. Sensible timescales are vital; they need to be challenging but not impossible to achieve. Unrealistic deadlines may prevent the project getting started, while an open-ended project may never reach completion. As discussed earlier, changes in culture, values, beliefs and attitudes do not happen overnight. Furthermore, winning over one colleague may be rather less time-consuming than changing the behaviour of the whole team, and drawing up a reasonable work schedule requires considerable thought and careful negotiation with those involved.

Reflection point seven: realistic timescales

• Is this the right time to start the project?
• What needs to be done?
• Can the project be divided into individual tasks?
• What order do tasks need to be completed in? Can some be undertaken simultaneously?
• How long will each task take?
• How much time are individuals able to allocate to the project within each working week? Does time out need to be negotiated?
• What are the key milestones? Can the project be staged or divided into manageable parts?

Gantt charts, as illustrated in Figure 3.5, are a useful means of representing the activities that need to be undertaken, their sequence and expected duration.

The timing of the initiative, given other events that are occurring within the environment, should be considered first. While there is rarely a perfect period in which to initiate a change in practice, undertaking too many changes at once or in quick succession is best avoided. The ability to

Key tasks	J	F	M	A	M	J	J	A	S	O	N	D
Undertake literature search	■	■										
Critically appraise literature		■	■									
Agree research questions				■								
Produce research proposal				■	■							
Submit proposal to ethics committee						■						

Figure 3.5 A simple Gantt chart for the first six months of a research project.

prioritize is an important skill that most nurses have and which needs to be drawn on in such situations.

The time elapsed between the introduction of a new idea and action is, however, also important. Too long and individuals lose interest, too short and people do not have time to adjust to the idea nor to express any concerns or needs they may have.

Evaluating and consolidating change

The means by which the change in practice or service delivery will be evaluated and consolidated should be built into the project plan and considered in the planning stages. However, as it is so easy to overlook, evaluation and the 'refreezing' stage of Lewin's (1951) model is given separate mention here.

Evaluation of a project can be undertaken from several perspectives and through both formal and informal means. Audit, questionnaires and surveys are useful. However, prescheduled and ad hoc meetings and feedback sessions also serve a useful purpose and may provide richer data. The approach chosen is dependent on the nature of the information required, with a combination of quantitative and qualitative approaches being most helpful.

Reflection point eight: evaluation

Outcomes

- Did the project achieve its objectives?
- What were the benefits for the patient/client?
- Were there any benefits for the professionals involved or for the organization as a whole?

Process

- Was the project well managed?
- Was it completed within the allocated timescale and budget?
- Did the process of change lead to any incidental benefits such as improved teamwork or communication?
- Will evaluation take place, prospectively, retrospectively or concurrently?

Leadership and change

Successful leaders inspire a shared vision, enable others to act, challenge the status quo, experiment, take risks and search for opportunities. However, they also lead by example, collaborate, recognize and celebrate the contributions of others (Kouzes and Posner, 1995; Girvin, 1998). These are all fundamental practices not dissimilar to those required of a successful change agent. Many (if not all) of the skills associated with successful leadership are therefore also required to promote growth and change in practice.

Conclusion

It is one thing to outline a simple programme of change and quite another to implement it (Pattison, 1996). Change rarely involves such an ordered sequence of events as that described here. Modifications to even the most well-constructed plans are often required. The timescales, process or even the end product of a project may require revision in the light of unexpected events. Careful planning and a systematic approach will increase the likelihood of success. However, the nurse practitioner needs to accept that change, while exciting, can be difficult to manage and is almost impossible to achieve alone.

References

Bernhard LA, Walsh M (1995) Leadership the Key to the Professionalization of Nursing. St Louis, Mo: Mosby.

Chin R, Benne KD (1985) General strategies for effecting changes in human systems. In: Bennis WG, Benne KD, Chin R (eds) The Planning of Change, 4th edn, pp22–45. New York: Holt, Rinchart & Winston.

Collinson G (1999) Ethical change. In: Hamer S, Collinson G (eds) Achieving Evidence Based Practice: a handbook for practitioners. London: Harcourt.

Covey S (1994) The Seven Habits of Highly Effective People. London: Simon & Schuster.

Earlam S, Brecker N, Vaughan B (2000) Cascading Evidence into Practice. Brighton: Pavillion Publishing and King's Fund.

Gillies, DA (1994) Nursing Management: A systems approach, 3rd edn. Philadelphia: WB Saunders.

Girvin J (1998) Leadership and Nursing. London: Macmillan.

Greene P, Elffers J (1999) Power: the 48 laws. London: Profile Books.

Huber D (2000) Leadership and Nursing Care Management. Philadelphia, Pa: Saunders.

Jones A, McDonnell U (1993) Managing the Clinical Resource – an action guide for health care professionals. London: Baillière Tindall.

Kitson A (1997) Developing excellence in nursing practice and care. Nursing Standard 12(2), 33–37.

Kouzes JM, Posner BM (1995) The Leadership Challenge: how to keep getting extraordinary things done in organizations. San Fransisco, Calif: Jossey-Bass.

Lewin K (1951) Field Theory in Social Sciences. New York: Harper.

Manion J (1998) Understanding the Seven Stages of Change. In: Hein EC, Contemporary Leadership Behaviour: selected readings. Philadelphia, Pa: Lippincott.

McPhail G (1997) Management of change: an essential skill for nursing in the 1990s. Journal of Nursing Management 5, 199–205.

Morris S, Willcocks G, Knasel E (2000) How To Lead A Winning Team. London: Prentice Hall.

Mullins L (1996) Management and Organisational Behaviour. London: Pitman.

NHS Centre for Reviews and Dissemination (1999) Getting evidence into practice. Effective Health Care Bulletin 5(1), 1–16.

NHSE (1998) Achieving Effective Practice: a clinical effectiveness and resource information pack for nurses, midwives and health visitors. London: Department of Health.

Pattison S (1996) Change management in the British National Health Service: a worm's eye critique. Healthcare Analysis 4, 252–258.

Perlman D, Takacs GJ (1990) The ten stages of change. Nursing Management 21(4), 33–38.

Rogers EM (1983) Diffusion of Innovations, 3rd edn. New York: Free Press.

Swage T (2000) Clinical Governance in Healthcare Practice. Oxford: Butterworth Heinemann.

Taylor B (1999) Personal change. In: Hamer S, Collinson G (eds.) Achieving Evidence Based Practice: a handbook for practitioners. London: Harcourt.

Upton T, Brooks, B (1999) Managing Change in the NHS. Buckingham: Open University Press.

Recommended reading

Morris S, Willcocks G, Knasel E (2000) How To Lead A Winning Team. London: Prentice Hall.

Mulhall A (1999) Changing Practice: the theory. London: Emap Healthcare.

NHSE (1998) Achieving Effective Practice – a clinical effectiveness and resource information pack for nurses, midwives and health visitors. London: Department of Health.

Scott CD, Jaffe DT (1997) Managing Organisational Change: a guide for managers. London: Kogan Page.

Upton T, Brooks, B (1999) Managing Change in the NHS. Buckingham: Open University Press.

CHAPTER 4

Breaking the boundaries

JULIE D'SILVA

Introduction

The prodigious challenges of provident healthcare in the UK in the 1990s and the growing consumer demands led many NHS trusts to create extended clinical roles for nurses. An important factor that aided this development was the publication in 1992 by the United Kingdom Central Council (UKCC) for Nursing and Midwifery and Health Visiting of its *Scope of Professional Practice* (UKCC, 1992), in which nurses were encouraged to further develop their roles. This publication advised nurses that they should access educational resources to ensure that they remained clinically competent practitioners (UKCC, 1992), placing the responsibility on the individual nurse to remedy deficits in knowledge which might prevent delivery of effective and appropriate care to patients and clients.

Other important factors that contributed to developing these new roles were waiting list issues. In 1991, the introduction of the Patient's Charter gave patients the right to be seen within two years of referral on to a waiting list. Targets set by the Department of Health to reduce the number of hours worked by junior doctors required that by the end of 1996 no junior doctors should work more than 72 hours per week.

The directive from the government that patients are to be seen within two weeks of being referred to the hospital by the general practitioner when they are suspected of having cancer will have an enormous impact on workloads, with waiting lists for routine referrals expected to rise significantly.

In response to these issues many trusts are creating new roles, with the nursing profession playing an active part in developing these roles.

The development of the clinical nurse practitioner roles was a natural progression for the clinical nurse, who saw the need for specialist roles in specific areas. The profession supported these changes in role with the introduction of 'The Scope' document, which encouraged nurses to expand their clinical roles (UKCC, 1992). The government went one step further to support professional bodies when the White Paper *The New NHS – Working Together* (DoH, 1998) introduced the concept of human resource strategy, which emphasized workforce planning, skills development, provision of managerial support and incorporated an overall aim to improve the quality of working life.

Following 'Agenda for Change', the new government recommendations for modernization and rationalization of the NHS pay scheme (DoH, 1999b), and the introduction of consultant nurse posts, a new career structure for nurses is unfolding. Experienced practitioners will be given the opportunity to advance their careers in practice, depending on responsibility, competence and performance. Career progression in this new role will develop through continuing education, professional development and personal planning to assess the level of practice required for the post holder.

Making a Difference (DoH, 1999a), a strategy produced by the Department of Health for England in an effort to promote the development of a clinical academic career for nurses and midwives, suggests that there should be:

- 'more flexible career pathways into and within nursing and midwifery education', with
- 'nurses taught by those with practical and recent experience of nursing'
- 'determination to enhance the status of those who provide practice-based teaching'.

This is welcomed by nurses wishing to expand their practice within the academic framework of university-based continuing education. It is also necessary to work within a framework for clinical practice to ensure consistent high-quality care for the patient, high clinical standards and improved risk management. Standards and clinical performance should be reviewed and updated regularly to guarantee competence and adequate performance, and to highlight training and development needs. Clinical governance has played a major role in this area and is a joint responsibility. All nurses must play their part in the team in which they work so that they can respond to their continuing professional development needs. Specific protocols and guidelines developed for the practice of the post holder should be implemented using a multidisciplinary team approach that takes into account research, new developments, legal requirements and national guidelines.

The British Society of Gastroenterology (BSG) has also produced guidelines against which standards in endoscopy units should be set, and has advocated that extended roles such as the nurse endoscopist should be considered (BSG, 1994). The guidelines were produced by a working party made up of professionals from specialist areas of gastroenterology and designed as a tool on which the practitioner can develop specific protocols for his or her own area. The reason the BSG produced these guidelines was because of the increasing interest and demand from both the medical and nursing professions for nurses to perform endoscopy, supporting initiatives to reduce waiting lists and developing fast-track clinics where certain cases would be seen more promptly. Legally, nurses can perform an endoscopy as long as the necessary training has been provided and they have the support of their trust, with adequate supervision provided by the consultant responsible, including careful patient selection to exclude high-risk patients. The BSG states that the required training for nurse endoscopy should follow the same regime as for the medical profession and should include attending a recognized course in endoscopy relevant to the type of procedure being undertaken and a module on anatomy and physiology. The nurse endoscopist should also continue with her education and maintain competence, supported by endoscopy courses and meetings relevant to her subject topic.

The Joint Advisory Group (JAG) for training and standards in gastrointestinal endoscopy across all specialities introduced specific guidelines for the endoscopist in 1999 (BSG, 1999), defining training and competency requirements. Units that provide training have to be approved by JAG. General practitioners, radiologists and nurse practitioners performing endoscopy are encouraged to register with JAG to ensure that standards of training are maintained to allow an opportunity for redress if standards do not appear to be maintained.

Extended practice

Differing roles

Clinical nurse specialist roles in the UK have developed over the past five years and it is important to remember that these roles should not result in the nurse specialist becoming a technician. It is therefore essential that the correct training is undertaken and the specific targets of the role are defined. It is better to clarify these roles before the post holder takes up the position; however, some roles evolve and new skills may become apparent as the role develops. It is advisable to have an established framework to build on. Nurses should not be appointed to a new post and be expected to work in isolation with no managerial and professional guidance or support.

Job titles

There are also many differing job titles, which should reflect the type of role undertaken, e.g. nurse practitioner, nurse specialist, clinical nurse specialist and nurse endoscopist, to name but a few. This can be rather confusing, as often there is not a clear understanding of the difference between job titles, and two practitioners doing similar roles may have different job titles. No definite job roles for expanded practice have been defined, so many nurses and managers have devised job titles to fit in with local interpretation and understanding of the title. The confusion surrounding job titles has been exacerbated by the misunderstanding of the differences between the roles. Often the managers writing the job descriptions are unsure of the responsibilities attached to the titles of nurse practitioner and clinical nurse specialist; therefore confusion has arisen. Changes will occur as laid down in the government document, *Making a Difference* (DoH, 1999a), which describes 'developing a modern career framework' to strengthen professional leadership and clarification of roles and responsibilities.

Job descriptions

Detailed job descriptions should be compiled to reflect the contents of any new post and should be regularly reviewed at individual performance appraisals with managers. The job description should take into consideration tasks that are actually performed, accountability, legal issues, support and appraisal. With the development and acceptance of a new post the volume of work will increase, making extra demands on time. It is essential that this is taken into account so that extra duties can be incorporated into the timetable and the practitioner does not overstretch herself. Once trained, the management of the practitioner should be reflected in the job description to ensure good accountability and supervision.

Management of roles

Depending on the type of role, it may be necessary to have more than one line manager:

- Business/Nurse manager – responsible for absence monitoring, annual leave, work rotas and professional nursing issues.
- Consultant/Supervisor – responsible for the management of clinical issues.

This may vary from trust to trust and according to job role.

It is essential that the nurse practitioner should work with both her nursing colleagues and other members of the multiprofessional team to monitor and improve the quality of care.

Clinical accountability varies from post to post and these issues need to be clarified by the post holder. In most instances, clinical management of the patient is likely to remain with the consultant, or a combination of the consultant and nurse, but not with the nurse alone. The consultant should act as the nurse's supervisor even when the nurse is trained and educated to the level required.

The General Medical Council (GMC) book *Professional Conduct and Discipline: fitness to practise* (1993) states:

Delegation of medical duties to nurses and others

The Council recognises and welcomes the growing contribution made to health care by nurses and other persons who have been trained to perform specialist functions, and it has no desire either to restrain the delegation to such persons of treatments or procedures falling within the proper scope of their skills or to hamper the training of medical or other health students. But a doctor who delegates treatment or other procedures must be satisfied that the person to whom they are delegating is competent to carry them out. It is also important that the doctor should retain ultimate responsibility for the management of these patients because only the doctor has received the necessary training to undertake this responsibility.

The nurse practitioner, however, should ensure she is competent in her role and mindful of the personal accountability she bears for her actions. She must be able to justify her clinical actions and decisions. She must also be aware of her limitations and able to identify what she is not in a position to do; this may be due to lack of practical skills or underpinning knowledge. In this instance, she should be able to identify means of remedying the situation if it is included in her remit and, if not, she should not be pressured into situations she is not qualified for.

Clinical governance

The introduction of the clinical governance initiative may have an impact on the way practitioners approach accepted professional standards and the quality of care delivered.

There are subsections under the umbrella of clinical governance covering clinical audit, risk management, continuing professional development, and research and clinical development. This is a formal team approach to improving the standards of care by using the four subsections to implement changes in practice if necessary.

Clinical supervision

Clinical supervision is a means of evaluating standards and offering support in clinical and professional development. Individual nurses are responsible for the safety of their practice and maintenance of their clinical competencies. 'For all practitioners in new roles, appropriate weight should be given to self assessment and peer group assessment where there is an available peer group, as well as the use of clinical supervision as a mechanism for safeguarding standards' (UKCC, 1992).

Many practitioners may have to go outside their own trust to find the appropriate supervision group because of the rarity of such posts. The main aim of clinical supervision is to offer support in clinical and professional development. It should provide opportunities for practitioners to discuss clinical issues with colleagues in order to reflect on their practice and, where necessary, make appropriate changes. It also offers to the practitioner who works in isolation some support and guidance from her peer group. The key benefits of clinical supervision are guidance, support and identifying skills, and it can be motivational. It can also help with identification of areas of poor or weak practice. Many practitioners do this informally by networking with colleagues during refreshment breaks at meetings and study days.

Nurse prescribing

Prescribing adds a further dimension to the role of the nurse practitioner. Nurse endoscopists are required to judge patients' specific needs in their area of expertise, ensuring patients receive holistic care from one practitioner. Some endoscopic procedures require the administration of sedation prior to the examination, and it would be defeating the object of the practitioner's role if she had to get a doctor to administer the drugs required to sedate the patient.

The Medical Defence Union (MDU) suggests in a summary of main recommendations from a final report of the committee looking at nurse prescribing that a UK-wide advisory body should be set up to assess submissions from professional organizations for suitably trained people to become independent or dependent prescribers. The advisory board would consider training and regulation as well as the clinical need. Once a group application was accepted individuals would be able to apply. The hope is that this would set standards of training, skills and competence (Parker, 1999).

This would be one way to develop nurse prescribing, but until such recommendations are achieved, nurses are working within clinical guidelines and administering drugs utilizing patient group directive criteria.

Personal reflection

Clinical practice

The need to develop a clinical nurse practitioner (CNP) role in the trust where I worked became evident due to the increase in demand for flexible sigmoidoscopy as a diagnostic test for patients presenting to their GPs with left-sided colonic symptoms. We decided the best way forward was a direct access route to the endoscopy unit. The implementation of this role was a joint decision by the multidisciplinary team.

Clinical nurse practitioner: flexible sigmoidoscopy for rectal bleeding/altered bowel habit

Flexible sigmoidoscopy has an increased role in the management of patients presenting with rectal bleeding or altered bowel habits. Due to growing waiting lists and consumer demands for a more efficient service, current clinical staffing and working practices were identified as inadequate, and had to be addressed.

Proposal

In an attempt to improve the service, the multidisciplinary team agreed that the appointment of a trained CNP would improve the service by providing a high standard of shared, informed decisions concerning the patients' care.

To bring about practice development in this area it was necessary to have the support of all concerned, therefore enabling co-ordinated planning and implementation of the CNP performing flexible sigmoidoscopy. Educational plans were discussed to identify what training was required and the best ways of achieving this. The team made a joint decision that the educational needs for this post were academic as well as practical, and it was decided that attendance at an external course was needed to fulfil the objectives.

Aims

• To improve the service by reducing waiting lists to enhance the quality of care the patient receives.
• To develop and implement protocols to be applied in the clinical area. Concise documentation is necessary to ensure high-quality clinical standards. All members of the team should be involved when preparing protocols and guidelines, as these will vary in different endoscopy units. National guidelines and legal requirements should also be taken into account.
• To audit and evaluate changes in practice to improve the service.
• To maintain personal development by obtaining knowledge, skills and experience necessary to the role.

Objectives

On developing the role of the CNP in clinical practice the following issues were addressed:

• The CNP will, in conjunction with the multidisciplinary team, produce written standards utilizing research-based practice.
• The CNP will access educational resources to remain a competent clinical practitioner and take steps to remedy any relevant deficits in order to effectively and appropriately meet the needs of patients and clients, as stated in the *Scope of Professional Practice* (UKCC, 1992).
• The CNP will develop an audit model to support innovation in practice.

Action plan

The multidisciplinary team formulated a business plan, which was presented to the clinical management team, outlining the need for a CNP in this area; this was accepted. It was agreed that the practitioner would develop specific skills in the area of flexible sigmoidoscopy for the detection of early colorectal cancer, and health education for patients suffering with irritable bowel disease, diverticular disease and inflammatory bowel disease. This would be achieved by providing advice to patients and promoting lifestyle changes where necessary. Standards of care and protocols were developed so the practitioner could act accordingly, thereby ensuring appropriate follow-up care of patients attending for flexible sigmoidoscopy.

Training was undertaken externally in the form of an English National Board (ENB) Colorectal Screening Course for Nurse Practitioners at Humberside College of Health, which is now part of the University of Hull.

On completion of training, nurses spent 12 months consolidating learning, gaining experience and confidence by working closely with the consultant supervisor. During this time further funding became available to support the development of the direct-access colorectal screening session for colorectal bleeding.

To enhance the service, further education modules have been undertaken in conscious sedation and therapeutic intervention during flexible sigmoidoscopy. Education and training is ongoing such that nurses successfully meet the assessment criteria to undertake all aspects of the nurse practitioner role in this speciality.

Summary of protocol

Practice guidelines are '... systemically developed statements to assist practitioner and patient decisions about appropriate health care for specific clinical circumstances' (Field and Lohr, 1992).

1   Prior to the setting up of the direct-access facility for colorectal bleeding, information and specific referral forms relating to the clinic were sent to all GPs in the area. A meeting was held with the GPs prior to the launch, explaining about the clinic and the referral criteria for accessing the clinic. Visits were made to practices that were unable to attend so that any questions or queries regarding the service could be addressed.

GPs refer patients via a specifically developed referral form to the consultant surgeon's secretary. Referrals are discussed and an appointment is made depending on the urgency of the referral. The consultant surgeon in question is the CNP's supervisor, and was throughout her training.

2   Indications for referral to this direct access facility are:

- rectal bleeding, particularly if recurrent or first-time bleed in elderly
- rectal bleeding with altered bowel habit
- rectal bleeding over the age of 40 years with a family history of colorectal cancer in first-degree relatives.

3   Referrals are prioritized; following appropriate selection criteria patients will be screened by the CNP, thereby reducing outpatient visits.

4   Prior to the procedure, patient-friendly information is sent to the patient, as well as a bowel preparation with instructions on administration. There is a contact telephone number for the endoscopy unit so any queries can be answered by staff trained in endoscopy, if required.

5   Not all patients require a barium enema. If from the referral letter it is felt that a barium enema will be required, then an oral bowel preparation will be sent with the appropriate instructions for use, and dietary requirements. Guidelines are in place so that the CNP can order barium enema if required.

6   After routine admission to the endoscopy unit the patient will be interviewed by the CNP and a set of specific questions will be asked regarding:

- medical history; specific questions are asked referring to rectal bleeding (Appendix 4.1)
- informed consent.

7   The procedure is performed without sedation unless specifically requested by the patient. A specific sedation module accredited by the ENB was undertaken externally at Humberside College of Health to enable the CNP to administer sedation prior to the procedure. A conscious sedation scale is used to ensure over-sedation does not occur. The amount of sedation administered is written on the procedure form and on a drug administration form.

8   Any abnormalities are identified and videoed or photographed for discussion with the supervisor.

9   Biopsies are taken of any abnormalities and sent to the laboratories for histological examination, with a copy of the report being sent to the consultant and the CNP.

10 Any difficulties relating to the procedure will be referred to the consultant supervisor immediately for guidance, advice and support. The consultant supervisor has an endoscopy list running concurrently with the CNP list.

11 Outcome is discussed with the consultant and further investigations and treatments are arranged for the patient before discharge.

12 On completion, a specific procedure form is completed (Appendix 4.2) by the CNP. She keeps a copy for audit purposes and the other copy goes into the patient's medical notes.

13 A letter will be sent to the GP and the patient with the results. If the results need explaining or if further investigations/treatment are required then an outpatient appointment will be arranged.

The introduction of a CNP in this area proved to be successful by:

- improving and maintaining high-quality care for patients presenting with colorectal bleeding
- reducing waiting lists for urgent referrals
- reducing the number of outpatient visits
- meeting consumer demands for an increased, more efficient service
- relieving pressure on clinical staffing.

The government proposal that everyone with suspected cancer will be able to see a specialist within two weeks of their GP deciding they need to be seen urgently, will put extra pressure on endoscopy units to see patients with suspected upper and lower gastrointestinal cancers. In preparing our business plan for the year 2000 we felt it was a necessary requirement to appoint a second full-time CNP to provide a faster, more efficient service.

Future developments

Public expectations and the context of care are changing; we are looking towards fast, efficient, convenient services. To achieve these standards there is a need to focus on certain priorities: improving health, strengthening services, providing prompt and effective care to achieve the best outcomes. There will be more opportunities for nurses to extend and develop their roles. They will play a more vital part in delivering care and using their skills to the full to improve access to nurse-led services and clinics. Developments in technology, e.g. telemedicine and telecare, will enhance screening programmes, making consultation, diagnosis and monitoring more efficient, and resulting in a higher standard of care and treatment. Data can be transmitted between different sites so expert advice and opinions can be sought more rapidly, saving time and resources, and improving care.

Nurse consultant posts will become established, providing new career opportunities for nurses. These posts will vary, depending on speciality needs and the service in which they are to be established. Consultancy posts will be developed for CNPs working in gastroenterology to deal with the increasing demands on the service and offer expert nursing practice. These posts will also provide an opportunity to improve services to bring them in line with government policies to improve healthcare for the general public. There will be more emphasis on education and training needs to develop new roles in practice.

Universities and NHS trusts, working together, are developing more appropriate specialist degree courses for practitioners in new roles to ensure the qualification is relevant for the specific clinical and academic skills required by the practitioner.

References

BSG (1994) The Nurse Endoscopist. Report of the BSG Working Party. London: British Society of Gastroenterology.

BSG (1999) Joint Accreditation Guidelines (JAG): recommendations for training in gastrointestinal endoscopy. London: British Society of Gastroenterology.

DoH (1998) The New NHS – Working Together: securing a quality workforce for the NHS. London: Department of Health.

DoH (1999a) Making a Difference: strengthening the nursing, midwifery and health visiting contribution to health and healthcare. London: Department of Health.

DoH (1999b) NHS Executive: Agenda for change. London: HMSO.

Field MJ, Lohr KN (1992) Guidelines for Clinical Practice. Washington, DC: National Abbey Press.

GMC (1993) Professional Conduct and Discipline: fitness to practise. London: General Medical Council.

Parker S (1999) Nurse prescribers – good for patients? Journal of the MDU 15(3).

UKCC (1992) Scope of Professional Practice. London: United Kingdom Central Council for Nursing, Midwifery and Health Visiting.

Appendix 4.1 Medical history: rectal bleeding.

HISTORY SHEET

RECTAL BLEED

COMMENCED . . . .

CONTINUOUS WITH EACH STOOL   YES   NO

INTERMITTENT . . . .

BLOOD

MIXED WITH STOOL . . . .

ON SURFACE OF STOOL . . . .

ON ITS OWN . . . .

MUCUS   YES   NO

BOWEL HABITS

NO. PER DAY . . . .

URGENCY   YES   NO

TENESMUS   YES   NO

ABDOMINAL PAIN . . . .

DEFECATION PAINFUL   YES   NO

OTHER

WEIGHT LOSS. . . . .   AMOUNT . . . .

ANAEMIA (IF CHECKED)   YES   NO

IF YES LAST H.B: . . . .

PREVIOUS HISTORY/INVESTIGATIONS

SIGMOIDSCOPY: BARIUM ENEMA:

SURGERY:

MEDICAL HISTORY

ANGINA/INFARCT   COAD/ASTHMA

DIABETES MELLITUS   ARTHRITIS/MUSCULAR/SKELETAL:

SIGNATURE   DATE

Appendix 4.2 Flexible sigmoidoscopy: procedure form.

PATIENT ID LABEL   ENDOSCOPIST   DATE

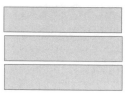

CONSULTANT REFERRED BY:

GENERAL PRACTITIONER:

SEX: MALE/FEMALE

INDICATIONS:

BOWEL PREPARATION

MICROLAX/FLEET/ORAL

RESULT: GOOD/POOR

DISTANCE OF INSERTION: CM

SEDATION

P/R EXAMINATION:

PATHOLOGY SEEN:

BIOPSIES TAKEN

TREATMENT/FURTHER INVESTIGATIONS REQUIRED:

FOLLOW-UP COLONOSCOPY: YES/NO

COMMENTS

SIGNATURE: DATE

CHAPTER 5

Evidence-based care, research and audit

MAGGIE GRIFFITHS

Introduction

The aim of this chapter is to explore the concept and developments of evidence-based nursing (EBN) and examine the use of research and audit in everyday practice. It will:

• outline the background to the development of evidence-based practice in nursing
• examine some definitions and provide information on how to access EBN resources
• discuss research and audit in everyday practice.

The second part of the chapter will provide some practical tips for the newly appointed practitioner.

Background to the development of evidence-based care in nursing

In 1972, the Briggs Report (DHSS, 1972) advocated that nursing should be a research-based profession with research underpinning nursing practice, nurse education and management. Prior to this, nursing practice had tended to be based more on tradition and ritual.

Over the past 25 years much nursing research has been carried out but difficulties remain in the implementation of findings and the links between research and practice. The reasons for the difficulties have been well researched, and strategies to overcome them will be discussed in the second part of the chapter.

The drive to develop evidence-based practice was also part of the wider NHS agenda. In 1991, the National Health Service (NHS) Research and Development (R&D) Strategy was launched. Its aim was 'to secure a knowledge based health service in which clinical, managerial and policy decisions are based on sound and pertinent information'.

In 1992, the United Kingdom (UK) Cochrane Centre was founded. This Centre forms part of an international network whose role is to prepare, maintain and disseminate systematic reviews of research on the effects of healthcare. The launch of the Cochrane Centre was followed by other funded national initiatives from the Department of Health, including medical and clinical audit and clinical effectiveness programmes for all healthcare professionals. The difficulty with this approach was that these initiatives were perceived by some practitioners and managers as being separate issues, rather than part of an overall approach to quality improvement.

In 1997 the Labour government was elected and the NHS was one of their priorities for reform and improvement. The publication of the White Papers *The New NHS: modern, dependable* (DoH, 1998a) and *A First Class Service, Quality in the NHS* (DoH, 1998b) continued the debate and outlined a modernization plan for the NHS. They were produced, in part, as a response to the major investigations that have been carried out in the NHS over recent years, which has dented public confidence in the service. These include the Bristol enquiry into cardiac surgery on babies (Smith, 1998) and the Kent and Canterbury hospitals cancer screening programme, where women were given incorrect results. What these enquiries demonstrated was a lack of appropriate systems and processes in place in all parts of the healthcare organizations to ensure the delivery of high-quality clinical healthcare, and an unhealthy organizational culture.

The White Papers emphasized the need to deliver high-quality, evidence-based healthcare by appropriately trained and updated practitioners and an NHS culture that was 'open' and less blame oriented. *A First Class Service* (DoH, 1998b) stated: 'There is concern when it is thought patients are being denied potentially beneficial new treatments. But a wider, if less reported, concern is the number of patients being denied proven treatments because of a delay by health professionals and managers in acting on published evidence. The time lag between research paper and bedside practice means many patients are being denied effective therapy.'

These consultation papers resulted in the Health Act 1999, which outlined the following main changes for the NHS:

- The establishment of clear national standards for services and treatments through National Service Frameworks (NSFs) and a National Institute for Clinical Excellence (NICE) whose role is to provide evidence on current best practice. NSFs have been produced for cardiac services, cancer, mental health, diabetes and the older person.
- Local delivery of high-quality healthcare, through clinical governance underpinned by modernized professional self-regulation and lifelong learning. The emphasis here is for the individual to be committed to lifelong learning and having access in the workplace to appropriate resources for updating their knowledge and skills.
- Effective monitoring of progress through a Commission for Health Improvement (CHI). The purpose of the CHI is to help the NHS in England and Wales assure, monitor and improve the quality of clinical care, by independently scrutinizing local clinical governance arrangements. More details on the CHI can be found on the Internet on www.chi.nhs.uk and NICE at www.nice.org.uk.

In July 2000 *The NHS Plan: a plan for investment, a plan for reform* was published which outlined a ten-year modernizaton plan for the NHS with targets and a strategy for how these changes would be achieved and care improved (DoH, 2000).

Clinical governance

Clinical governance is 'a framework which helps all clinicians, including nurses, to continuously improve quality and safeguard standards of care' (RCN, 1998). The components of the clinical governance framework include systems for clinical audit, complaints, litigation, risk management and quality improvement programmes. Sometimes these systems are in place – the difficulty is that they are not always linked and therefore lessons are not learned from risk incidents or patient complaints and practices changed to improve patient care.

The consultation document for quality in the new NHS (DoH, 1998b) set out frameworks for improvements in healthcare through clinical governance. Every healthcare organization is now expected to have a clinical governance committee. This committee is a subgroup of the trust board, and the trust board will receive reports from it on a regular basis. The trust is also required to submit an annual report on its progress in clinical governance to the NHS Executive. These changes will help to bring about a change in the culture of the NHS to become more open and less blame oriented. It is hoped that this will demonstrate openness to the staff, patients and families and help rebuild public confidence in the NHS.

Part of the reason for this emphasis on evidence is linked to the debate within the NHS on the financing of cost-effective and appropriate healthcare. The funding issues are outside the remit of this chapter, but different ways to fund healthcare in the 21st century, due to the development of technological advances and demographic changes, continue to tax the minds of politicians and managers both here and abroad.

Before discussing evidence-based nursing practice, it may be helpful to define some associated terms to aid clarity.

- Evidence-based medicine: 'the conscientious, explicit and judicious use of current best evidence in making decisions about the care of individual patients. The practice of evidence based medicine means integrating individual clinical expertise with the best available external evidence from systematic research' (Sackett et al., 1996).
- Clinical effectiveness: 'clinically effective practice is what results when practitioners use the best possible health care practices to achieve the best possible patient health outcomes, and rather than replacing standard setting and audit it includes them; the standards and criteria reflect the 'best practice' and audit is used to promote the implementation and evaluation of practice against those standards of best practice' (RCN, 1996).
- Research: a systematic investigation undertaken to discover facts or relationships and reach conclusions using scientifically sound methods (Hockey, 1996). 'Research is a planned, logical process. Research may be undertaken for the purpose of analysing relationships between events, or for predicting outcomes' (Clifford, 1997).
- Clinical audit: a clinically led initiative which seeks to improve the quality and patient outcome of patient care through structured peer review whereby clinicians examine their practices and results against agreed explicit standards and modify their practice where indicated (NHS Executive, 1996).
- Evidence-based practice: 'an approach to decision making in which the clinician uses the best evidence available, in consultation with the

patient, to decide upon the option which suits that best' (Muir Gray, 1997). The conscientious, explicit and judicious use of current best evidence, based on systematic review of all available evidence – including patient-reported, clinician-observed and research-derived evidence – in making and carrying out decisions about the care of individual patients. The best available evidence, moderated by patient circumstances and preferences, is applied to improve the quality of clinical judgements (McGibbon et al., 1995; National Centre for Clinical Audit, 1997). This definition emphasizes the use of evidence, the patients' views and clinical expertise.

- Evidence-based nursing: evidence-based nursing can be thought of as a branch of the work of Archie Cochrane and David Sackett, who led the development of evidence-based medicine.

'In a nutshell, the aim of evidence based nursing is to make it easier to include current best evidence from research in clinical and healthcare decisions' (Flemming, 1998). This approach has been operationalized in a five-stage process:

- Information needs from practice are converted into focused, structured questions.
- The focused questions are used as a basis for literature searching in order to identify relevant external evidence from research.
- The research evidence is critically appraised for validity and generalizability.
- The best available evidence is used alongside clinical expertise and the patient's perspective to plan care.
- Performance is evaluated through a process of self-reflection, audit or peer assessment (Flemming, 1998).

As Closs and Cheater (1999) report 'the expertise which patients (or their families) can contribute to decisions about care is made explicit in this approach and is an important element ... patients with long term health problems ... accumulate considerable expertise in the self-management of their conditions, which should be taken into account in decisions about their care'. This is an important point for patients and clients with whom the gastroenterology team will have contact. It recognizes the involvement of patients and the clinical expertise of practitioners, not just the use of evidence in a 'sterile' way. It also counters the criticism that is sometimes levelled at evidence-based practice, in general that it is a 'cookbook' approach to healthcare and does not allow sufficient emphasis on the individual patient.

It can be argued that by disregarding rituals it enables the practitioner, as part of the multiprofessional team who are all using an evidence-based approach, to decrease the level of overlap and duplication. This will enable more focused and effective care to be provided to the patient and his or her family.

There are both opportunities and challenges for practitioners in the development of evidence-based practice. If the nursing evidence is lacking it may be worth noting Kitson's (1997a) advice. She reports: 'Where best evidence does not exist, one should be encouraging a much more systematic approach to the description and use of interventions.' As she points out, for relatively young professional groups, of which nursing is one, the amount and quality of research evidence to draw on may be fairly limited compared with older, more established professions. However, when considering this issue, it may be worth bearing in mind an American study by Aiken (1990), who reported that in every multi-hospital study on mortality in the US and Canada, nursing was among the important factors that explain variation in deaths between hospitals.

Exercise

- What is your organization doing to implement EBP?
- Is there an appropriate strategy that you can use to help in your area?
- What resources are available, e.g. people, IT, financial?
- How can you access them?

How to access information on evidence-based practice and research findings

There are five main sources of information available to the practitioner, depending on what type of information is required.

1 Textbooks

These are mainly used as texts for information that is unlikely to change or are basic texts for the subject area.

2 Journals

These can vary from research publications to more general journals discussing professional issues. They may be uniprofessional or multidisciplinary.

3 Bibliographic databases

Two of the most popular are CINAHL and Medline. CINAHL, the Cumulated Index to Nursing and Allied Health Literature, is produced by CINAHL Information Systems and their website address is www.cinahl.com/ It is a general database for nurses and other healthcare professionals from the USA. It includes citations from more than 650 English-language journals. It also contains an extensive bibliography of related articles.

Medline is produced by the US National Library of Medicine and covers all areas of healthcare. Embase is another database. An article by Burnham and Shearer (1993) provides a description of three databases and compares the results of the searches for specific clinical topics.

Pubmed and Internet Grateful Med (www.nlm.nih.gov/databases/freemedl.html) are two free services from the US National Library of Medicine.

4 Distilled and consolidated information sources

As McGibbon and Marks (1998) note, 'despite the peer review process, not all research studies published in journals are methodologically sound and some may be more sound than others'. In 'distilled' information sources, the information has been reviewed and assessed for its quality and only those studies that have been considered the best are presented. EBN and Medicine are of this type of information source.

Sometimes there may be conflicting evidence on particular topics and consolidated information sources have been developed to examine the evidence. This may be due to the research design and the methodology used. In a systematic review, these differences are examined and attempts made to reconcile them by examining the primary studies. The UK Cochrane Centre produces systematic reviews and involves all disciplines that participate in healthcare together with users of the NHS. It is dependent on groups of individuals with interest in the same clinical topics meeting to review the literature.

The Cochrane Library (www.cochrane.co.uk/) includes four databases.

- The Cochrane Database of Systematic Reviews contains the full text of more than 300 systematic reviews and protocols of more than 300 planned or ongoing systematic reviews.
- The UK NHS Centre produces the Database of Abstracts of Reviews of Effectiveness (DARE) for Reviews and Dissemination at the University

of York. It contains more than 1500 records of international systematic
reviews.

- The Cochrane Review Methodology Database contains references to
  articles on the methods and approaches to systematic review.
- The Cochrane Controlled Trials Register is a database of trial
  information.

There is a charge to access some databases.

5 The Internet

There is a great deal of choice on the Internet for all types of information.
The following may be helpful to start with.

- The Centre for Evidence-based Nursing based at the University of York
  (www.york.ac.uk/inst/crd)
- Department of Health R&D home page (www.doh.gov.uk/research/
  index.htm).

Exercise

There is a lot to choose from. The following questions may be helpful in
deciding priorities:

- Are there some textbooks that you need to buy as an investment? Are
  they available on CD-ROM?
- What journals do you need access to?
- Are they available locally?
- Are they research-based or on general topic areas?
- Are they peer-reviewed by experts in the field of gastroenterology?
- Are they national or international publications?
- What journals do you need to look at from other healthcare professions?
- Do you need to brush up search skills for the databases?
- Can you access the Internet?

With all this evidence, how is 'best' evidence arrived at and what happens
if the evidence conflicts? There need to be some criteria to judge it against.
Closs and Cheater (1999) argue: 'Reliable knowledge has three crucial
attributes: it must be in the public arena and it must be both consensible
(understood) and consensual (agreed) (Ziman, 1978, p6) ... furthermore it

must be presented in such a way that it is widely and uniformly understood (consensibility).'

Muir Gray (1997) also looked at strength of evidence and the way they compared. He identified five types.

- Strong evidence from at least one systematic review of multiple well-designed randomized controlled trials.
- Strong evidence from at least one properly designed randomized controlled trial of appropriate size.
- Evidence from well-designed trials without randomization, single group pre–post, cohort, time series or matched case control studies.
- Evidence from well-designed non-experimental studies from more than one centre or research group.
- Opinion of respected authorities based on clinical evidence, descriptive studies or reports of expert committees.

Effective use of EBN will make practice more appropriate, timely and acceptable to the patient, the team and the organization. Because of the emphasis on the need for evidence-based care from clinicians, the patients and the NHS Executive, the time has never been better to develop skills in EBN. Taking a systematic approach to searching for evidence can result in better time management. Using Flemming's approach can save time in a pressurized role by not becoming buried in too much paper!

Once the research evidence has been gathered, it is vital that the practitioner recognizes and develops strategies to deal with the implementation of research findings. There needs to be clarity about how evidence is used by all members of the multiprofessional team.

In 1997, Hunt undertook a major study of the problems of introducing research findings and confirmed the difficulties involved in change. However, she was able to implement rational changes by involving nurse teachers, ward sisters/charge nurses and managers in teams to identify the problems using the research literature and change practice as appropriate. This led Hunt to argue that as great an effort is needed to implement change as is required to discover it.

Change will be a continuing factor in healthcare delivery and the practitioner will be involved in it, in his or her own practice and in the organization where he or she works. As Kitson (1997b) notes, 'change has to be seen as a normal component of any care delivery system'. The practitioner therefore needs to be aware of the issues that affect successful change management. There have been other papers reporting on the profession's progress in implementing research findings and the problems associated with it. The indications are that cultural, organizational and personal factors prevent the use of nursing research in practice (Closs and Cheater, 1999; Funk et al., 1995; Watt. 1993).

Other reports note the need for support when implementing changes (Alexander and Orton, 1988). It is worth bearing this work in mind, as it can be very trying to deal with the difficulties and the frustrations of some of these issues. Appropriate support, both for the individual nurse specialist and the ward team who may be implementing the change alongside the rest of their busy agenda, is vital. To facilitate this the nurse specialist will require an understanding of how teams work and how they can be influenced; who in the team are the opinion formers; who need to be convinced first before the other team members will follow.

Initiating research can be difficult and time-consuming. Collaboration with other staff and the resources of a local university with a health studies department can be invaluable in developing joint projects and influencing the research agenda. If this is done, the likelihood of the research sitting on a shelf unused is minimized.

If planning an initiative or a research bid, discussion about implementation and what resources are needed to make this happen are required. For example, it may be appropriate to include a sum for implementation of the findings.

Audit

Simple records will make audit easier and provide information and activity data to enable an analysis of referrals, trends, etc. An audit of service is needed to demonstrate the effectiveness of role and resources and the link to the individual's personal development plan. This plan will demonstrate the commitment to lifelong learning and fit with the clinical governance framework.

The use of clinical audit, together with the practitioners' audit programme, can demonstrate the impact on patient outcomes, for the individual patient and for the organization. For example, access to a gastroenterology nurse may prevent admission to hospital and save money in ensuring the use of appropriate appliances. This can lead to a reduction in the number of people attending the outpatients department.

It also needs to be remembered that record keeping can be tiresome. It is important to be clear about the following:

- What records are needed?
- Who is to do the record keeping?
- Simplification of existing sources of information.
- What help/resources are available to help and support audit?

Exercise

- What standards will you audit against?
- What audit method will you use?
- How will your findings be analysed/fed back/used to change practice?

Conclusion

Clarke (1999) argues that 'health care is at heart a human orientated practice' and as humans are different, this diversity should be reflected in the evidence gained and valued. To illustrate this she records the following anecdote.

During the Second World War a young doctor named Archie was taken captive and spent the rest of the war a prisoner. He served as a camp doctor and one day was attending a severely wounded young Soviet soldier. He recounts the day:

> The ward was full, so I put him in my room as he was moribund and screaming and I did not want him to wake the ward. I examined him. He had obvious gross bilateral cavitation and a severe pleural rub. I thought the latter was the cause of the pain and screaming. I had no morphia, just aspirin, which had no effect, I felt desperate. I finally, instinctively sat down on the bed and took him in my arms, and the screaming stopped almost at once. He died peacefully in my arms a few hours later. It was not the pleurisy that caused the screaming, but loneliness. It was a wonderful education about the care of the dying. I was ashamed of my misdiagnosis and kept the story a secret.
>
> (Cochrane and Blythe, 1989, p. 82)

The doctor was Archie Cochrane, one of the founding fathers of evidence-based medicine. This anecdote highlights that evidence is important but so is clinical expertise, the ability to recognize patient's needs, intuition and instinct, and listening to patients and other colleagues who may have the knowledge, expertise and evidence we lack.

For this part of the chapter the author was given a free hand to write a vignette, an interview or a description of an initiative or whatever would be useful to the practitioner. I decided to offer a practical list of things that I wish someone had told me when I became a specialist nurse. The list is in no way exhaustive and has been developed with insights from other nurse specialists with whom I have had the privilege to work. This is our contribution to you and hopefully you will find it helpful in making your job even more enjoyable.

- Being a nurse specialist does not mean you are a cross between Florence Nightingale and Superman/woman. People will still have problems that you will not be able to solve singlehandedly.
- Never assume that what is obvious to you is obvious to other people, whether they are healthcare professionals, patients or carers.
- Time taken planning your service will not be wasted. Once you have a clear idea it will make it easier to explain how the service is going to start and develop. Remember that some of the people you will be explaining your service to may not have a clinical background or your knowledge and insight, so you may need to explain in more detail.
- Work out how you are going to manage your workload. Some useful questions that you may want to think about:

  - Are you going to have referral criteria?
  - Are you going to see all referrals yourself?
  - What about urgent patients?
  - How are your patients going to be followed up?
  - How are you going to educate and develop other staff?
  - When are you going to make time for you personally and professionally?
  - Where will your base be in relation to your patients?
  - Is there parking available for your car, bike or other form of transport?
  - The nurse specialist has four components to the job: clinical, research, management and education. How are you going to split your time and resources?
  - What are your communication skills like? Good communication, written and oral, is critical.
  - Who have you seen and what has happened to them? Keeping simple records of this will aid audit and demonstrate how your time is allocated and the outcomes of your practice.
  - Do you need to brush up your skills on assertiveness or time management?
  - Are you politically aware and do you know the people of influence in your organization?
  - How are you going to gain organizational support?

- Indicators of care: do you need them? What are you going to use, and why?
- How are you going to ensure that your practice links to the clinical governance framework in your organization?
- What is the organizational culture and how are you going to influence it?

References

Aiken LH (1990) Charting the future of hospital nursing. Image 22, 72–74

Alexander M, Orton H (1998) Research in Action. Nursing Times 84(8), 38–41.

Burnham J, Shearer B (1993) Comparison of CINAHL, EMBASE and MEDLINE databases for the nurse researcher. Medical Reference Service Quarterly 12, 45–57.

Clarke JB (1999) Evidence-based practice: a retrograde step? The importance of pluralism in evidence generation for the practice of health care. Journal of Clinical Nursing 8, 89–94.

Clifford C (1997) Nursing and Health Care Research, a skills based introduction (2nd edn). New Jersey: Prentice Hall.

Closs SJ, Cheater FM (1999) Evidence for nursing practice: a clarification of the issues. Journal of Advanced Nursing 30 (1), 10–17.

Cochrane AL, Blythe B (1989) One Man's Medicine. British Medical Foundation for AIDS, London.

DHSS (1972) Report of the Committee on Nursing. Cmnd 5115. London: HMSO.

DoH (1998a) The New NHS: modern, dependable. London: The Stationery Office.

DoH (1998b) A First Class Service, Quality in the NHS. London: Department of Health.

DoH (1999) Review of the Nurses, Midwives and Health Visitors Act: Governemtn response to the recommendations. London: Department of Health.

DoH (2000) The NHS Plan. London: Department of Health.

Flemming K (1998) Asking answerable questions. Evidence Based Nursing 1(2).

Funk SG, Tornquist EM, Champagne MT (1995) Barriers and facilitators of research utilisation. Nursing Clinics of North America 30, 395–407.

Hockey L (1996) The nature and purpose of research. In: Cormack DFS (ed) The Research Process in Nursing, 3rd edn. London: Blackwell.

Hunt J (1997) Towards evidence based practice. Nursing Management 4(2).

Kitson A (1997a) Using evidence to demonstrate the value of nursing. Nursing Standard 11(28), 34–39

Kitson A (1997b) Developing excellence in nursing practice and care. Nursing Standard 12(2), 33–37.

McGibbon KA, Marks SM (1998a) Searching for the best evidence. Part 1: Where to look. Evidence-Based Nursing 1(3), 68–70.

McGibbon KA, Marks SM (1998b) Searching for the best evidence. Part 2: Searching for CINAHL and Medline. Evidence-Based Nursing 1(4).

McGibbon KA, Wilczynski N, Hayward RS, Walker-Dilks CJ, Haynes RB (1995) The medical literature as a resource for health care practice. Journal of American Society for Information Science 46, 737–742.

Muir Gray JA (1997) Evidence-based Health Care. How to make health policy and management decisions. Edinburgh: Churchill Livingstone.

National Centre for Clinical Audit (1997) Glossary of Terms Used in the NCCA Criteria for Clinical Audit. London: NCCA.

NHSE (1996) Clinical Audit in the NHS. Using Clinical Audit in the NHS: a position statement. Leeds: NHS Executive.

RCN (1996) Clinical Effectiveness. A Royal College of Nursing Guide. London: Royal College of Nursing.

RCN (1998) Guidance on Clinical Governance. London: Royal College of Nursing.

Sackett DL, Rosemberg WMC, Gray JAM, Haynes RB, Richardson WS (1996) Evidence-based medicine: what it is and what it isn't. British Medical Journal 312, 71–72.

Smith R (1998) All changed, changed utterly: British medicine will be transformed by the Bristol Case. British Medical Journal 316, 1917–1918.

Watt GCM (1993) Making research make a difference. Health Bulletin 51(3), 187–195.

Ziman J (1978) Reliable Knowledge. An exploration of the grounds for belief in science. Cambridge: Cambridge University Press.

Further reading

Clifford C (1997) Nursing and Health Care Research, a skills based introduction, 2nd edn. Hertfordshire: Prentice Hall Europe.

Sackett DL, Richardson WS, Rosenberg W, Haynes RB (1997) Evidence-based Medicine: how to practise and teach EBM. Edinburgh: Churchill Livingstone.

CHAPTER 6

Risk management and assessment

PAULINE HUTSON

Introduction

Risk management is one way of reducing identified risks to the lowest level of acceptability. This is a corporate response to all potential errors within an organization and is not confined to either clinical or non-clinical hazards. A new approach to risk management has recently been initiated as part of the main framework of clinical governance. In addition to carrying the ultimate responsibility for resources, chief executives now carry responsibility for the quality of service within each trust. The concept of risk management must therefore play a key role in the assurance of quality care.

This can have no greater relevance than to the role of the nurse practitioner, who has potentially increased the exposure to risk by advancing clinical practice. The nurse practitioner in gastroenterology is perhaps even more vulnerable, due to the huge diversities within the role.

This chapter aims to consider a strategy for risk management within the endoscopy environment. It is not meant to be definitive, but will stimulate a proactive approach to the subject. It will encroach on issues discussed in other chapters, but this will be in the context of risk and is necessary to incorporate all aspects of care.

The origins of risk management

The initial impetus for risk management has been governed by a growing need to reduce litigation and complaints. This has become an increasing concern for the UK during the past decade and a major worry for clinicians in the US over the past two decades (Vincent, 1995). This has harnessed the rather negative view of risk management as nothing more than a protection for the hospital against claims. There is speculation that this approach will be seen as merely 'paying lip service' to an initiative that will not produce a reduction in claims and litigation (Dimond, 1998). A more positive view is that it provides a fundamental approach to improving quality of care.

Certainly the key turning point to risk management began with the introduction of Crown Indemnity by the government in 1990 and the subsequent withdrawal of Crown Immunity from health authorities in 1991. This had an enormous impact on healthcare in general, as the responsibility for damages arising from clinical negligence claims was devolved to the relevant health authority. In addition, the Health and Safety Executive could now introduce fines and penalties directly to NHS trusts.

In response to these initiatives a proactive approach to risk management has been adopted by most NHS trusts. Corporate strategies, which take account of generic issues such as staff training in movement and handling, and health and safety, are now considered mandatory. While this may provide evidence of good practice, it can only serve to represent the foundations for additional risk management strategies.

The principles of risk management

Much of the work relating to the principles of risk management is based on the report by Merrett Health Risk Management Limited, who in 1992 were commissioned by the NHS to undertake pilot studies within several NHS trusts. The aim of this exercise was to produce a manual that would provide guidance on risk management to healthcare organizations. The experience of risk managers outside the NHS was used in the compilation of the document, which means that much of the work is health and safety focused. However, the basis of the risk management process as illustrated in the document provides a useful tool for reference (NHS Executive, 1994).

Risk identification

Results from the NHS Executive pilot studies have resulted in four main modules on which to focus risk identification:

- risks that have a direct impact on the patient
- risks that have an indirect impact on the patient

- health and safety
- organizational risks.

Risks may encompass any one of the modules or may be interrelated. For instance, if there is no regular, mandatory training for staff in cardiopulmonary resuscitation techniques, there is a risk that could impact directly on patient care. If, however, there is no evidence of a corporate strategy to initiate training, then the risk is also organizational.

Identification of risks can therefore be a potentially dissatisfying and frustrating business, particularly if huge costs or changes are envisaged as a result. It may be tempting to ignore issues that may ultimately identify further risks, particularly if the implications for doing so involve other clinical teams. All too often the impetus for change has to come from corporate management, who may not fully comprehend the justification for such measures.

Many trusts these days have introduced a risk management group whose main aim is to address operational issues and initiate a proactive culture. Other methods of highlighting risks can be through formalized risk assessment forms. Health and Safety Departments are usually more than willing to guide staff through the use of such forms and to provide further advice.

Risk analysis

Evaluating the severity of the risk is perhaps more difficult. Most identified risks in the NHS are difficult to quantify, and defining the probability of recurrence may be too subjective for accuracy. The use of incident forms within most trusts provides some quantifiable data to assist in the identification and analysis of risks. It is possible, through such records, to build up a strategic picture of organizational shortfalls. Key areas are also highlighted in order that improvements in training and staff awareness can be implemented.

Risk control

The fundamental part of the process of managing risk is to take control. The NHS Executive guidelines (NHSE, 1994) ask four questions to consider how the risk can be controlled:

- How can it be eliminated – prevention?
- How can it be avoided – avoidance?

- How can it be made less likely – acceptance?
- How can it be made less costly – acceptance?

The most attractive proposition would be to adopt techniques that would eliminate the risk. For example, the risk of aspiration pneumonia in a patient receiving both sedation and throat spray is eliminated by administering one drug only. However, by comparison, the potential complications of the sedated endoscopy patient would not exist at all if sedation was not administered. While the elimination of this risk is impractical, this type of risk can be reduced to some degree by using a robust system of selective sedation, in addition to safe patient monitoring.

These examples are routine, everyday decisions that most people would not consider under the title of risk management and emphasize the fact that controlling risks is not the sole responsibility of the organizational hierarchy.

In some instances, managing an identified risk has to be through risk acceptance. This is perhaps where the managerial and organizational function has most input. Accepting a risk but rendering it less likely to happen is one of the pinnacles of hospital management. National guidelines such as the NMC *Guidelines for Records and Record Keeping* (NMC, 2002) are supported in NHS trusts by local policies and procedures. These measures serve a dual purpose. Risks are reduced down to the absolute minimum and there is an agreed benchmark against which all incidents can be compared.

Attempting to make a risk less costly involves a comparison of potential losses against plans to cover the risk through insurance. The endoscopy department is little different from any other major department in that the cost of equipment is high and additional maintenance can be a drain on resources. A budgetary response, which takes account of the age of equipment against the cost of a warranty cover, may be appropriate to ensure that equipment is constantly updated and available. Unfortunately, in many endoscopy centres in the UK, the need for endoscopy exceeds resources (Sobala et al., 1991). This can have a detrimental effect on endoscopes, which are constantly rotating through disinfecting machines and wash cycles. In addition, the workload of the endoscope is increased if other scopes are out of action for repair work. The correct handling and use of such equipment can play a large part in reducing repair work to a minimum. Unfortunately, good practice cannot totally eliminate the risk of breakdowns and a clever juggling act is required to balance the justification for insurance costs against the potential cost of repairs.

Risk funding

Risk funding is, however, an integral part of any department, irrespective of the type of equipment in operation. Budgetary planning is one way of controlling risks, but unfortunately there is no bottomless pit of money and budgets in most trusts are stretched beyond desirable limits. This poses the question of prioritization, which requires an objective stance, as most people will consider that the needs within their own department are most important. The NHS Executive suggests a simple technique to use when attempting to prioritize risks:

frequency × severity = risk exposure

Categorization of frequency and severity into low, medium and high terms needs to be used as a benchmark within each organization. However, while this may reduce subjectivity to some degree, the accuracy of probability is questionable.

Application of risk management

The remit of the gastroenterology nurse practitioner is extremely diverse and will involve nurses from a variety of backgrounds. There will be those who have worked in the endoscopy unit for years, and therefore risk management in this area will have become second nature. However, there will be some who have had very little endoscopy experience and, as such, are entering a new and very different environment.

In addition, there will be those who consider risk management as being at the heart of health and safety policies and fail to acknowledge the concept as being a fundamental part of nursing care. Indeed, the standards of care for patients are so closely related to risk management that the difference is often difficult to detect.

This chapter will therefore address the application of risk management first to the care of the patient within the gastroenterology environment and second to the endoscopy unit. The central focus in both cases will be to develop a strategy of risk assessment that supports the nursing care of the patient and considers how risks can be eliminated or at least reduced to a minimum.

The patient

Patient assessment

Pre-assessment of a patient prior to an endoscopic procedure is the starting point for reducing associated risks to the lowest possible level. To gain the most from this exercise, it needs to be carried out accurately, documented clearly and by appropriate trained personnel.

It is important to understand that the information gained from the assessment is likely to impinge on all aspects of risk management for that patient. The nurse practitioner must be aware that information from the patient regarding drug allergy, past medical history and family background may be inaccurate, if the patient is particularly distressed or anxious. Patients often fail to mention medical interventions that they perceive as being totally unrelated to their gastrointestinal complaints. A hip prosthesis may be taken for granted by a patient regardless of the risk from careless positioning on the endoscopy couch. Caution may be warranted if the use of diathermy is required on patients with pacemakers, and antibiotic cover may be required as a prophylactic measure on patients with a history of endocarditis (Stafrace, 1998).

If the pre-assessment is being carried out by endoscopy nursing staff and not by the nurse practitioner, the observation of the patient's anxiety levels can only be related second-hand. The nurse practitioner must then make decisions regarding treatment based on written information only, as an assessment of anxiety levels once the patient is in the endoscopy room may not reflect accurately levels of anxiety during the pre-assessment interview. It would be unfair and unwise to ask the patient to reconfirm the essential facts as it would only increase the patient's distress.

The BSG recommendations for standards of sedation and patient monitoring during gastrointestinal endoscopy state that patients 'at risk' include those classified as American Society of Anesthesiologists (ASA) grades III–V, the elderly and those with heart disease, cerebrovascular disease, significant lung disease, liver failure and jaundice, acute gastrointestinal bleeding, anaemia, morbid obesity and shock (BSG, 1991). However, while this list seems fairly comprehensive it fails to acknowledge patients who are heavy smokers, have high alcohol intake or who may be extremely anxious.

Therefore an assessment of the patient must be taken in collaboration with an assessment of procedural risk. The BSG guidelines (1991) suggest that cardiopulmonary complications predominate in gastroscopy examinations, whereas perforations and bleeding are common during colonoscopy examinations. These risks are potentiated by additional factors and the nurse practitioner must acknowledge therefore that, on occasion, a referral to a more senior and experienced clinician is a sign of good risk management and should never be viewed as failure.

Informed consent

The Patient's Charter (1995) provides explicit information about the rights and expectations of patients. In addition, it clearly states that explanations of proposed treatment and any associated risks are to be provided. Unfortunately, the capability of the patient to fully understand the implications of and reasons for a procedure may be difficult to assess, particularly in the elderly. This is when the risks associated with gaining informed consent become apparent. The BMA (1995, p14) states that:

> it is the personal responsibility of all health professionals proposing to treat a patient, to determine whether the patient has the capacity to give a valid consent.

The first hurdle for the nurse practitioner therefore involves assessing the capacity of the patient to consent to or refuse permission for the procedure (Hall Harris, 1995). Faulder (1985) considers the three main elements for consent. The first two elements are based on the understanding that the relevant information is made available, including the right to say 'no' to treatment. The third element is based on two rules: the patient must know that she is giving it and must understand what it involves.

In 1999, the BSG issued a document providing 'Guidelines for Informed Consent for Endoscopic Procedures'. This is a comprehensive guide for all endoscopists, providing clear information relating to the law and informed consent. In terms of risk assessment, the nurse practitioner needs to be aware of the two key examples of case law, which are outlined in the document as being the most pertinent. The first refers to *Bolam* v *Friern Hospital Management Committee* (1957) 1 WLR 582, which states:

> he or she must act in accordance with a responsible body of relevant professional opinion. (p5)

It is worth mentioning here that there are relatively few nurse practitioners currently established in the UK and therefore it is likely that 'a responsible body of relevant professional opinion' would be that of a group of doctors working in gastroenterology.

The second refers to the case of *Sidaway* v *Board of Governors of Bethlem Royal Hospital* (1985) AC871, which states:

> that a decision on what degree of disclosure of risks is best calculated to assist a particular patient to make a rational choice as to whether or not to undergo a particular treatment must primarily be a matter of clinical judgement, however a judge might come to the conclusion that the disclosure of a particular risk was so obviously necessary that no reasonably prudent medical man would fail to make it. (p6)

The BSG has attempted to address this issue in part by recommending the use of specific consent forms, which clearly state the potential complications of endoscopic procedures. These have been based on the premiss that a patient should be told of adverse events of a minor nature if there is an incidence of 10 per cent, and serious events with an incidence of 0.5 per cent (BSG, 1999).

It is questionable whether more patients will refuse treatment as a result of new guidelines. The UKCC *Guidelines for Professional Practice* (1996) clearly state that the right to refuse consent must be respected; however, it would not be unreasonable to involve other members of the healthcare team to ensure that the patient is fully informed of the consequences. In addition, a summary of discussions should be documented in the patient's records.

Clearly, there is a risk of carrying out an endoscopic procedure on a patient who has not fully understood the implications. Most nurse practitioners will have been placed in the situation where the patient has asked for a nurse to explain what the doctor meant, despite the fact that the consent form may already have been signed. There is a suggestion that nurses will have far less of a problem treating the patient as an autonomous decision maker, as they have developed from a background which is not governed by paternalism and beneficence (Cook, 1992). Instead, the nurse practitioner has the continued support of the UKCC in advocating for patients who they feel have not been fully informed (UKCC, 1989).

In addition to assessing the risks when gaining patient consent, the nurse practitioner may be presented with further difficulties if the patient attempts to withdraw consent once the procedure has commenced. This is largely determined by the patient's tolerance of the procedure if full informed consent has been established prior to the event. Constant reassurance may sometimes be sufficient to calm a patient who has become agitated and distressed. However, there will be those who panic and may indicate that they wish to have the scope withdrawn. The decision to withdraw the scope is then left to the nurse practitioner. Depending on the clinical indications for the procedure, the justification for withdrawing the scope may be at odds with acting in the best interest of the patient, as there is a high chance that the patient will refuse to go through with the procedure again. If there is any risk that the patient will cause harm to himself, the endoscopy staff or indeed the endoscope, then there must be no doubt that the procedure should be terminated. If, however, there is a chance that stopping the procedure for a few minutes to clarify the patient's wishes and to explain the consequences of terminating

Table 6.1. Key points to consider when obtaining informed consent

When obtaining informed consent the patient must understand:
• the nature of the proposed procedure
• the reason for the procedure
• the benefits of the procedure
• the risks and complications of the procedure
• alternatives to the procedure
• the nature of anaesthesia or sedation to be used

Source: BSG (1999)

the procedure may calm the patient sufficiently to complete the procedure, then informed consent will have been restored.

Key points of the informed consent process as identified by the BSG (1999) are listed in Table 6.1.

Conscious sedation

There is a clear element of risk associated with conscious sedation of the endoscopy patient. Once sedation has been administered, the nurse practitioner is undertaking a dual role of sedationist and endoscopist. The BSG guidelines for 'Standards of Sedation and Monitoring during Endoscopy' (1991) provide recommendations to reduce these risks.

It is useful to bear in mind when reading the document, that this was written prior to the development of nurse-administered sedation. While this does not alter the concept of the guidelines, it may be prudent for the nurse practitioner to adopt additional measures to those proposed, such as the use of a conscious sedation scale. This provides a documented account of the patient's sedation experience. Clark (1994) introduced five variables to benchmark the assessment:

• emotional affect
• level of consciousness
• physical reaction to discomfort or pain
• variation in vital signs
• degree of amnesia.

Assessment of the patient continues throughout the procedure and the scoring system on discharge reflects three degrees of sedation: under, over or optimal.

The use of such a scale can be crucial to support essential clinical monitoring. While the need for pulse oximetry, blood pressure monitoring and oxygen saturation cannot be overemphasized, there is a danger that endoscopy staff rely too heavily on quantitative data. The results of an audit on the safety, staffing and sedation methods of gastrointestinal endoscopy in two regions of England (Quine, et al., 1995) caused enough concern to raise questions regarding the correct usage of pulse oximetry by endoscopy staff. Some units had monitors set to alarm at 85 per cent desaturation or lower, despite the fact that the clinical signs of cyanosis are rarely evident at this level. Charlton (1995) states that the use of pulse oximetry is considered to be mandatory by anaesthetists and it is equally accepted that oxygen saturation should not be permitted to fall below 90 per cent.

The siting of the monitoring probe must provoke further consideration. When measured on the distal phalanges, oxygen saturation levels can be severely affected by hypovolaemia, hypothermia, severe peripheral vascular disease, Raynaud's disease or high-dose vasopressors, all of which can cause vasoconstriction (Messina, 1994). While the ear lobe may be a more suitable area to ensure accurate readings, the lateral position of the endoscopy patient and the intervention of the nurse at the head of the patient during upper gastrointestinal endoscopy could easily dislodge the probe.

The risks of conscious sedation may be equally exacerbated if the probe is attached to the patient at the same time as sedation is administered. This disallows the advantage of establishing a baseline reading. A study by Hinzmann et al. (1992) identifed that the nurse was able to intervene sooner as a result of knowing baseline saturation levels and therefore was able to effect positive outcomes and reduce the risk of hypoxaemia.

The additional advantage of pulse oximetry when administering sedation is that it provides a clinical indication of appropriate dosage. The recommendations from the BSG state that the minimum dose of all drugs must be considered as standard practice. Drug protocols written at local level should preclude any alternatives. However, titrating the dose over several minutes may provide additional protection for the patient against over-sedation.

The use of supplemental oxygen for all sedated endoscopy patients remains a controversial issue. However, the BSG guidelines clearly state that supplemental oxygen should be administered to patients 'at risk'. Studies relating to the administration of supplemental oxygen have highlighted additional factors that may exacerbate hypoxaemia, particularly during upper gastrointestinal endoscopy. The experience of the endoscopist and subsequent length of procedure (Lavies et al., 1988), endoscope diameter (Lieberman et al., 1985) and sedation with midazolam (Bell et al., 1987) were all found to have a significant effect on oxygen saturation levels.

Table 6.2. Key points to consider in the management of a patient receiving conscious sedation

- If sedation is indicated, consider the suitability of each patient on individual assessment
- Ensure all essential resuscitation equipment and drugs are readily available in the endoscopy area
- Ensure that at least one qualified endoscopy trained nurse is monitoring the patient's condition throughout the procedure
- Establish a baseline reading of pulse oximetry before administering sedation
- Consider the use of supplemental oxygen, taking account of all relevant factors
- Titrate the dose of sedation in order to keep dosage to an absolute minimum
- Consider the use of a conscious sedation scale in addition to clinical monitoring
- Intravenous cannulae should be left in situ until full recovery has been established

Consideration of all known factors has to provide the framework for the nurse practitioner to assess the risks when administering sedation. In addition, the level of skill and experience from endoscopy nursing staff has to be that of at least one qualified nurse trained in endoscopic technique and dedicated to the care and monitoring of the patient. It is the responsibility of both the endoscopist and the nurse in charge of the area to ensure that equipment and drugs necessary for resuscitation are immediately available.

Reversal agents specific to the drugs being administered by the nurse practitioner should be immediately available for emergency use and should be subsequently included within the protocol for the nurse prescribing. The use of an intravenous cannula, which remains in situ until the patient is fully recovered, should be considered standard practice.

Key points to reduce risks associated with conscious sedation are listed in Table 6.2.

Exercise 1

A patient attending the endoscopy unit for an upper gastrointestinal endoscopy has requested sedation. She has a history of ischaemic heart disease and a previous myocardial infarction.

- What are the risks of administering sedation to this patient?
- What risks are you going to discuss with the patient prior to undertaking the procedure?
- What monitoring equipment would you use on this patient?
- How would you minimize the potential risks of administering sedation to this patient?

Drug protocols

In 1997, in response to the recommendations outlined in the 1996 White Paper *Primary Care: delivering the future*, a review of prescribing, supplying and administration of medicines was inaugurated. The main aim was to make greater use of the skills and experience of various professions working within primary and secondary care. The review team was chaired by Dr June Crown, President of the Faculty of Public Health Medicine, and work focused on the development of a legal framework to determine how health professionals could undertake new roles with regard to the prescribing, supply and administration of medicines. The key legislative requirements are set out in the Medicines Act 1968, which, if breached, renders a person liable to criminal prosecution.

The specifics of the report, however, will not exonerate the nurse practitioner if the impact of the drugs being administered is not fully understood. In addition, illegibility of drug charts, failure to document dosages accurately or carelessness in checking the dose given will almost certainly result in litigation.

Drug interactions

The drugs used by the nurse practitioner will depend on the procedure being undertaken and the drug protocol, which will have been previously negotiated at local level. The risks associated with each drug will have been discussed and the nurse practitioner should understand fully potential side effects and complications. In addition to information available in drug protocols, the BSG recommendations for standards of sedation and patient monitoring during gastrointestinal endoscopy (1991) and the Royal College of Surgeons' *Guidelines for Sedation by Nonanaesthetists* (1993) provide clear information on the risks associated with patient sedation and, as such, should be available to the nurse practitioner.

The Royal College of Surgeons is keen to point out that the responsibility for risk assessment lies clearly with the sedationist and cannot be devolved to referring consultants or GPs. The key to success, therefore, must be in the initial assessment of the patient's suitability for sedation and the endoscopist's experience to cope with potential difficulties.

The use of benzodiazepines is the most common choice for sedation and an assessment of the patient prior to administration is crucial. This should take account of the age of the patient, the weight of the patient and any coexisting medical conditions, such as cardiac, renal or hepatic failure. Titrating the dose is always recommended and the patient's response, in addition to careful monitoring of pulse and oxygen saturation, should be observed. Full sedation will have been reached when the patient is drowsy, has some degree of slurred speech but is still able to respond to commands. Occasionally the administration of a benzodiazepine can produce severe hypoventilation and hypoxia (Lieberman et al., 1985). This may be more prevalent during upper gastrointestinal endoscopy, due to the physical presence of the endoscope in the pharynx.

One of the most commonly used benzodiazepines is midazolam, which can cause a change in respiratory pattern, with a decrease in tidal volume but an increase in frequency. As a result, the abdominal contribution to respiration becomes depressed, although the thoracic contribution is preserved (Dundee et al., 1984). The elimination half-life of midazolam is 1.5 to 3.5 hours in healthy subjects, but this can be prolonged in the elderly or obese.

The use of an opioid in addition to a benzodiazepine will potentiate the risk of adverse cardiorespiratory complications. There is evidence that a major drug interaction between the two types of drugs exists and studies have demonstrated that benzodiazepines are increased in potency as much as eight times, when given with an opioid such as pethidine (Ben-Shlomo et al., 1990). The doses of both drugs therefore should be reduced when administered together. The opioid should be given first and an appropriate length of time should be allowed before the benzodiazepine is cautiously titrated.

Antagonists to reverse the effects of benzodiazepines (flumazenil) and opioids (naloxone) must be available (Royal College of Surgeons, 1993). The use of antagonists should not be regarded as a solution to the risk management of sedation, and the associated risks when administering such drugs should be regarded with equal respect. The duration of the effect of the antagonists is less than with benzodiazepines and opioids, and therefore careful monitoring of the patient after administration should be employed until all possible effects of the sedation have subsided. The dose of the antagonists should be titrated over several minutes until the desired level of consciousness has been achieved. If the antagonist is administered too quickly the patient may become agitated and anxious.

All patients who have received sedation should be continuously monitored during the recovery period, and discharge from the unit will vary depending on the age and health of the individual. Adequate discharge information should emphasize the dangers of driving and operating machinery for at least 12 hours post-procedure.

Many patients, particularly those having an upper gastrointestinal procedure, will not require sedation. The use of local pharyngeal anaesthesia in these patients is generally adopted but should not be considered in conjunction with sedation, due to the increased risk of aspiration. In most units, patients are not allowed to eat and drink for one hour after administration and should be warned of possible numbness of the tongue or bucosal membrane to decrease the danger of biting trauma.

Record keeping

The use of risk management as a strategy for reducing litigation and complaints can have no greater emphasis than the consideration of accurate documentation. Tingle (1997) states: 'Medical and nursing records can win or lose a case.'

Any extension of role will inevitably create an increase in documentation relating to patient care and, as such, the risks associated with recording accurately, objectively and consistently are increased. The *Standards for Records and Record Keeping* produced by the UKCC in 1993, provide a comprehensive benchmark for all nurses and trusts. However, since the publication of the document, the Audit Commission continues to report on the ritualistic nature of record keeping in nursing and the lack of clear, relevant information.

The surge in nurse practitioner posts over recent years has highlighted a growing need to integrate care within the multidisciplinary team in order to avoid the scenario whereby each group of professionals plans its own aspect of care. This has resulted in the development of multidisciplinary care pathways, which provide clear directions agreed by all health professionals, specifying key events, tests and assessments in an appropriate order (Wilson, 1996). The development of care pathways for the gastroenterology nurse practitioner can provide a clinically based standard, which incorporates protocols, policies and practice guidelines. While ritualistic record keeping and duplication by other professional groups can thus be avoided, there is a danger of using a care pathway automatically. The individual needs of all patients must be taken into account, irrespective of the routine nature of proposed treatment, and any deviations or additions should be clearly recorded.

The use of shared records is becoming increasingly popular, whereby all health professionals involved in the care of the patient use the same reporting tool. This enhances collaborative working and provides an accurate chronology of events. A local framework for recording in this manner is recommended, in order that clinical audit can be processed. In addition, a clear indication of each health professional's identity must be evident.

Both the Data Protection Act 1984 and the Access to Health Records Act 1990 allow patients the right of access to their own health records. The UKCC has upheld this principle but is keen to point out to all practitioners that suitable terminology and careful consideration of language in all documentation is therefore paramount. The use of computer records is increasing, particularly for endoscopy recording. While the use of computer technology reduces the risk of litigation as a result of illegibility, the potential to record all aspects of a patient episode must be available within the software. Standards for signing reports and identification of the healthcare professional should not differ, irrespective of the methods used for documentation.

Exercise 2

A patient complains that the nurse practitioner gave an inadequate explanation following investigations for irritable bowel syndrome.

• How will you prove what information was given to the patient?
• Are there clear written protocols to support your treatment and advice for this condition?
• Did the patient receive written information relating to his condition, which would support and reiterate oral advice? Did you document that this had been given to the patient?
• How would you handle this complaint?

Communication

Poor communication in the NHS is one of the main causes of patient complaint and therefore forms a key area for clinical risk management (East, 1995). The development of nurse-led clinics in gastroenterology over recent years has lessened some of the professional barriers that nurses faced in the past when questioned by patients regarding their progress. However, this widening remit within the extended role has brought with it further problems, and academic courses that focus on issues such as breaking bad news reflect this change in culture.

Communication with the primary care teams has also increased with the advent of nurse-led clinics. Direct links between GPs and nurse practitioners have evolved, as patient referrals are dealt with and subsequent treatment proposed. Unfortunately the legislation to support the service is often lacking within the remit of the nurse practitioner and as a result, a great deal of time is spent contacting referring doctors.

Documentation of telephone conversations between nurse practitioners, patients and GPs is paramount to this service, and a systematic method of filing such records should be incorporated.

Continuity of care by the nurse practitioner from initial assessment through to an endoscopy procedure and follow-up improves communication, as information regarding treatment becomes less fragmented. Working in collaboration with the patient means that enough time is given for questions to be asked and, more importantly, for the answers offered to be comprehensible. Difficulties may arise because of the practitioner's perception of what is comprehensible, as the gap between the lay person and the health professional can vary enormously. Patients are easily distracted by questions that they find embarrassing but which are readily accepted by healthcare professionals.

Fear of litigation may influence decisions about how much information to give, particularly relating to the potential risks of treatment. It is tempting to discourage patients from asking questions which practitioners may feel uncomfortable in answering. A robust system of recording the information given to patients and relatives will devalue any claims of miscommunication. The use of good information leaflets to support oral communication will increase the potential for patients to understand treatment and conditions.

The risks relating to communication and record keeping are extremely similar. The key to controlling these risks includes clear, unambiguous documentation which includes every aspect of care, including relevant communication between patient, relatives and the multidisciplinary team. In addition, a robust system of record keeping which allows the potential for audit is paramount. Beckmann (1996) states: 'Let everyone know what you are thinking, planning and doing because surprises have no place in patient care.'

The endoscopy unit

Equipment

The safety of the patient in any hospital setting is the responsibility of all health   professionals, and the maintenance and correct use of all equipment is fundamental to a safe passage of care. A defined system of reporting equipment malfunction/failure should be evident within every NHS trust and it is the responsibility of every manager to ensure that all staff are fully aware of this process.

The Medical Devices Agency (MDA) is an Executive Agency for the Department of Health whose main role is to ensure that appropriate standards of quality and performance are met and that they comply with the Directives of the European Union. Incidents reported to the MDA are investigated and, where appropriate, action is taken to inform other users of potential hazards. An adverse incident is defined by the MDA as:

> an event which gives rise to, or has the potential to produce, unexpected or unwanted effects involving the safety of patients, users or other persons (MDA, 1999).

Reporting an incident to the MDA is not limited to equipment failure in the device itself, but includes:

* instructions for use
* servicing and maintenance
* locally initiated modifications or adjustments
* user practices, including training
* management procedures
* the environment in which it is used or stored
* incorrect prescription.

Once a report has been submitted, the equipment should be taken out of service and retained for further investigation. If appropriate, all readings of settings, switches, gauges and indicators should be included in the report, in addition to the usual critical incident information. Discussions with the Adverse Incident Centre may be required if the equipment is contaminated, and provision to inspect the equipment on site may need to be arranged.

Appropriate healthcare personnel should be aware of any hazard notices distributed by the MDA and relevant equipment should be taken out of service until it has been rendered safe for further use. The role of the MDA is crucial in developing standards of patient and staff safety. While clinical governance has highlighted the need for a comprehensive audit of adverse outcomes, a 'no blame culture' should be advocated, in order that incidents are analysed objectively and a systematic approach to improving subsequent outcomes is thus initiated. Moss (1995) suggests that risk management and clinical audit are complementary, not alternative, programmes relating to quality of care.

Endoscopic accessories

Concern about the reuse of endoscopic accessories was raised in 1998 by the BSG. The report was prompted by the Medical Devices Agency

Bulletin (MDA DB 9501) in 1995, which questioned the practice of reusing endoscopic accessories, irrespective of manufacturers' guidelines. As the legal liability for reprocessing equipment was subsequently transferred to organizations, a working party was set up to consider suitable recommendations for gastroenterologists, trusts, endoscopy units and manufacturers, with regard to these issues.

Accessories are classified into three groups:

- reusable – can be reused following appropriate cleaning, disinfection or sterilization. Reuse may not be unlimited and records should be kept of the number of times the equipment has been reprocessed. A system of checking that the equipment is still functional prior to use should be evident.
- single-use – mainly reflects low-cost items. Concern has been raised since the working party report that these should be labelled 'single patient use', as the term single-use indicates that each time the equipment is used, it should be discarded, even if the procedure it is being used for is incomplete and reuse would be on the same patient.
- reusable/single-use – the 1995 MDA bulletin gave clear requirements for the reprocessing of single-use items, which inferred that stringent technical requirements would be required to ensure the integrity and safety of each processed item.

As a result of the worries relating to the legal and regulatory position of the use of endoscopic accessories, the BSG working party made the following recommendations:

- Reusable accessories should be used where appropriate cleaning and sterilization procedures are bacteriologically sound.
- The manufacturers' advice must be taken for reusable accessories, and the accessories must be inspected before each cleaning cycle and immediately prior to use.
- Single-use items must not be reused unless the instructions in MDA DB 9501 are strictly followed.
- Manufacturers should work with users to issue appropriate advice on cleaning/disinfection/sterilization.

It is worth mentioning here that although the nurse practitioner in gastroenterology may work in the endoscopy unit only on a sessional basis, the responsibility for correct use of accessories or indeed any other equipment cannot be avoided. Knowledge of cleaning and disinfection techniques should be sought and management policies relating to the reuse of equipment should be known. Using defective or worn equipment will inevitably make a procedure more difficult and may ultimately damage the scope.

Infection control

Appropriate disinfection of endoscopes should eliminate any risk to the patient from cross-infection. However, methods employed to eliminate this risk should take account of staff health in relation to exposure to the chemicals used in the process. Both elements of risk cannot therefore be confined to the remit of endoscopy staff, and the nurse practitioner, along with all gastroenterologists, should be aware of local and legislative documents relating to the decontamination of endoscopes.

The MDA produced a document in 1996(a) (MDA DB 9607) which assessed the risk of transmission of micro-organisms to an individual patient being dependent on one of the following factors:

- the type of endoscopic procedure undertaken
- the micro-organisms present in any previous patient's secretions
- the effectiveness of the method used to reprocess the endoscope
- environmental recontamination of the endoscope during or after processing
- the susceptibility of the patient to infection.

The overall risk of infection following endoscopy is relatively low. Endoscopes used in upper and lower gastrointestinal endoscopy are deemed non-invasive as they are not invading sterile cavities and, as such, can be decontaminated using high-level disinfection. Inadequate decontamination procedures will result in the transmission of any organism present in patient secretions. Clear instructions on the decontamination of endoscopes following use on patients with viruses such as HIV and HBV are provided by relevant manufacturers of disinfection materials and should be supported by local policies advocated by infection control departments.

A BSG Working Party Report was published in 1998, which reviewed various disinfection agents and provided further recommendations for cleaning and disinfecting endoscopes. One of the key reasons for the publication of this document was that the legal occupational exposure level for glutaraldehyde, the most widely used disinfectant, had been reduced.

Trusts were therefore finding it increasingly difficult to comply with the Health and Safety at Work Act of 1974 and the Control of Substances Hazardous to Health Regulations 1988 (revised 1994). As a result, manufacturers have spent a great deal of time and money in attempting to produce a suitable alternative to glutaraldehyde that can provide adequate disinfection without undue risk to equipment or staff.

A collaborative decision on which disinfectant to use within an endoscopy unit is generally made after discussion with gastroenterologists, infection control departments and endoscopy unit managers, and much will depend on the type of disinfection machines in use. Regular meetings with endoscopy unit managers and endoscopy users provide an opportunity to review any reported incidents of cross-infection and to ensure that all members of the endoscopy team are continually informed of any changes in practice. The cleaning of endoscopes is an integral part of the endoscopy patient episode and yet in a study of staff attitudes towards the cleaning and decontamination of endoscopes (Foss and Monagan, 1992), 86 per cent of physicians and 30 per cent of nurses were unaware of the incidents of cross-infection.

For those nurse practitioners who are unfamiliar with the endoscopy environment, it is worth mentioning here that personal health and safety may be compromised if insufficient attention is paid to the type of disinfecting agent used in the endoscopy unit.

Although disinfection machines are housed in areas away from patients, all staff who regularly work within the endoscopy environment should be aware of the policy for dealing with a chemical spillage and, equally, should be trained in its implementation.

Electrosurgery

Although the use of electrosurgery will be limited within the remit of the nurse practitioner, a brief mention of associated risks is warranted. High-frequency current in monopolar electrosurgery flows from an active electrode through the patient's body to a neutral electrode, i.e. the patient plate. The current generates warmth in the body tissues, which rises proportionally to electrical resistance in the tissue and to the square of current density (Erbe, 1998).

The positioning of the patient plate is therefore critical to reduce the risks of electrosurgery to an absolute minimum. The electrical resistance to heat is higher in fat, and the plate should therefore be placed in an area where muscle is more predominant. Electrical contact will be impaired in the presence of excessive hair or scar tissue. In addition, the area of skin should be dry and the patient plate should not be positioned over a prosthetic joint.

Power settings should be kept to a minimum, and if an increase in power is required, this should be raised gradually until the desired effect is evident. A crucial point here is that the smaller the surface area, the greater the heat, which is particularly relevant to the use of snares, which can exceed temperatures of 100°C.

Relevant operating manuals for electrosurgical units should be available in all endoscopy units and the nurse practitioner should ensure she is familiar with the settings and operation of the unit prior to use.

Latex allergy

In 1996(b), the MDA published a bulletin that considered potential problems posed by latex sensitization in the healthcare setting (MDA DB 9601). This was updated in 1998, and more pressure was placed on managers to establish local policies relating to the justification of using powdered gloves (MDA SN9825). Although it is recognized that the starch powder is not an allergen itself, the protein residue in latex attaches to the starch and acts as a carrier, which can cause respiratory allergic reactions through surface or airborne transmission.

There will be a few patients who enter the hospital setting unaware of having a latex allergy. Suspicion should always be raised if a patient presents with a history of non-systemic allergic reactions such as contact urticaria, dermatitis, eczema and asthma (Brown, 1999). In addition, the MDA reports on the probability of such patients being sensitive to avocado, chestnuts or bananas.

The presence of latex in other products is perhaps more worrying than in the context of glove usage. A huge variety of hospital equipment contains latex products and each department should therefore have initiated a latex-free store of equipment, which can be immediately available for patients with a known allergy. The possibility of an allergic reaction should be considered in all patients who suddenly develop unpredictable symptoms, such as rhinitis, conjunctivitis, wheezing, throat tightness or asthma. The use of resuscitation equipment may be required, as the condition can result in anaphylaxis and death, in severe cases.

Exercise 3

Within the endoscopy environment, consider the measures that you would adopt when dealing with a patient who has a known latex allergy.

- Are there written guidelines within the department for the management of the sensitized patient?
- Is there latex-free equipment immediately available within the department?
- Are the appropriate drugs readily available to deal with an anaphylactic reaction?
- Would this patient be appropriate for the nurse practitioner to endoscope?

Manual handling

Irrespective of previous clinical experience, the nurse practitioner in gastroenterology will be familiar with the legislation associated with manual handling. However, an assessment of risks is paramount to the health and safety of all staff. *The Code of Practice for the Handling of Patients* (RCN, 1993) provides a framework based on the task, the patient, the environment, the equipment and the handlers. However, it should be pointed out that risks are not confined to the movement of patients around the department, but should be considered when positioning the height of equipment for ease of access, in particular the examination couch and the television monitor.

Exercise 4

Consider the manual handling issues associated with a clinically obese patient requiring a flexible sigmoidoscopy.

- Which type of bowel preparation should be considered, taking account of ease of administration and effectiveness?
- Is a patient hoist available within the endoscopy unit, if required?
- Would a patient commode provide easier access to toilet facilities? Is there a suitable area for the patient to use the commode if necessary?
- Do all patient transfer trolleys have a height adjustment mechanism?

Bowel preparation

The nurse practitioner undertaking endoscopic examination of the lower gastrointestinal tract needs to be aware of the risk factors associated with preparation of the bowel. A pre-assessment of the patient's potential for carrying out adequate bowel preparation in the home environment should have been undertaken through the referring physician. In addition, clear, written instructions on self-administration are crucial and the inclusion of a telephone contact number for advice or reassurance is desirable. The side effects of colonic lavage can include nausea, abdominal cramps, bloating, pain, dizziness and vomiting, and the age or medical history of the patient may suggest that hospital admission for bowel preparation would be advisable in order to reduce associated risks.

Hydration during purgation is a key issue and instructions on fluid intake need to be uncomplicated. The ingestion of large volumes of fluid are necessary with some osmotically balanced polyethylene glycol-based electrolyte solutions which irrigate the whole gut in a few hours (Bartram, 1994). Unfortunately, while the volume of fluid content in the bowel does not compromise a colonoscopy procedure, it is inappropriate if radiological investigation is required, as the viscosity of the barium reduces the capacity for mucosal coating.

The use of much smaller volumes of oral preparation, however, has been reported as preferable to patients. Vanner and colleagues (1990) report improved patient tolerance with oral sodium phosphate preparations. Unfortunately, raised levels of serum phosphate have been recorded, and patients with congestive heart failure, ascites or renal failure should be considered at risk.

The use of bowel preparation inserted via the anal route is indicated for sigmoidoscopy procedures; however, patient compliance should be considered if this is to be administered in the home environment. This type of preparation is unsuitable for patients with evident active bleeding, severe diarrhoea or ulcerative colitis.

The type of bowel preparation offered to patients is usually determined by the gastroenterologist's preference. However, the nurse practitioner performing the lower gastrointestinal procedures remains responsible for ensuring that an effective and clear examination of the bowel has been achieved. The risk of not recognizing neoplasms obscured behind small particles of faecal matter is increased by inadequate bowel preparation (Cohen et al., 1994).

Appropriate documentation is essential if a full view of the bowel has not been possible. Updating and reviewing existing bowel preparation with gastroenterologists may be necessary if examinations are compromised.

Conclusion

This chapter has explored the concept of risk management within the diversity of the gastroenterology nurse practitioner's role. In whatever setting the nurse practitioner may be based, the principles of risk management remain unchanged. A proactive approach to the reduction of risks must take account of quality, resources, legislation and audit. It must be undertaken within an organizational philosophy but should be managed appropriately within the multidisciplinary team. Good communication, both internal and external to clinical management teams, is essential to develop and sustain an effective risk management system.

References

Bartram CI (1994) Bowel preparation – principles and practice. Clinical Radiology 49, 365–367.

Beckmann JP (1996) Nursing Negligence. London: Sage Publications.

Bell GD, Reeve PA, Moshiri M, Morden A, Coady T, Stapleton PJ, Logan RFA (1987) Intravenous midazolam: a study of the degree of oxygen desaturation occurring during upper gastrointestinal endoscopy. British Journal of Clinical Pharmacology 23, 703–708.

Ben-Schlomo I, Abd-El-Khan H, Ezry J, Zohar S, Tverskoy M (1990) Midazolam acts synergistically with fentanyl for induction of anaesthesia. British Journal of Anaesthesia 64, 45–57.

British Society of Gastroenterology (1991) Recommendations for standards of sedation and patient monitoring during gastrointestinal endoscopy. Gut 32, 823–827.

British Society of Gastroenterology (1998) Report of the Working Party of the Endoscopy Committee of the British Society of Gastroenterologists on the reuse of endoscopic accessories. Gut 42, 304–306.

British Society of Gastroenterology (1999) Guidelines for Informed Consent for Endoscopic Procedures. http://www.bsg.org.uk

British Medical Association (1995) The Older Person: consent and care. London: BMA.

Brown K (1999) Care of the latex sensitive patient in theatre. British Journal of Theatre Nursing 9940, 170–173.

Clark BA (1994) A new approach to assessment and documentation of conscious sedation during endoscopic examination. Gastroenterology Nursing 15(5), 199–203.

Charlton JE (1995) Monitoring and supplemental oxygen during endoscopy. British Medical Journal 310, 886–887.

Cohen SM, Wexner SD, Binderow SR, Nogueras JJ, Daniel N, Ehrenpreis ED, Jensen J, Bonner GF, Ruderman WB (1994) Prospective, randomised, endoscopic – blinded trial comparing precolonoscopy bowel cleaning methods. Diseases of the Colon and Rectum 37(7), 689–696.

Cook T (1992) The nurse and informed consent. Senior Nurse 12(2), 41–45.

Dimond B (1998) Clinical risk management: is it just a sham? British Journal of Nursing 7(14), 813.

Dundee JW, Halliday NJ, Harper KW, Brogden RN (1984) Midazolam: a review of its pharmacological properties and therapeutic use. Drugs 28. 519–543.

East J (1995) Aspects of clinical documentation. British Journal of Healthcare Management 1(14), 716–718.

Erbe Medical UK Ltd (1998) NESSY, the Neutral Electrode Safety System for Increased Safety in Electrosurgery. Erbe Germany.

Faulder C (1985) Whose Body Is It? The troubling issue of informed consent. London: Virago Press.

Foss D, Monagan D (1992) A national survey of physicians' and nurses' attitudes towards endoscope cleaning and the potential of cross infection. Gastroenterology Nursing 15, 59–65.

Hall Harris C (1995) Issues and trends in nursing. In: Deloughery GL (ed) Legal Aspects of Nursing. St Louis, Mo: Mosby.

Hinzmann CA, Budden PM, Olson J (1992) Intravenous conscious sedation use in endoscopy: does monitoring of oxygen saturation influence timing of nursing interventions? Gastroenterology Nursing 15, 6–13.

Lavies NG, Creasey T, Harris K, Hanning CD (1988) Arterial oxygen saturation during upper gastrointestinal endoscopy: influence of sedation and operator experience. American Journal of Gastroenterology 83(6), 618–622.

Lieberman DA, Wuerker CK, Katon RM (1985) Cardiopulmonary risk of esophagogastroduodenoscopy role of endoscope diameter and systemic sedation. Gastroenterology 88, 468–472.

Medical Devices Agency (1995) MDA DB 9501 The Reuse of Medical Devices Supplied for Single Use Only. London: MDA Adverse Incident Centre.

Medical Devices Agency (1996a) MDA DB 9607 Decontamination of Endoscopes. London: MDA Adverse Incident Centre.

Medical Devices Agency (1996b) MDA DB 9601 Latex Sensitisation in the Health Care Setting (Use of Latex Gloves). London: MDA Adverse Incident Centre.

Medical Devices Agency (1998) MDA SN 9825 Latex Medical Gloves (Surgeons' and Examination) Powdered Latex Medical Gloves (Surgeons' and Examination). London: MDA Adverse Incident Centre.

Medical Devices Agency (1999) MDA SN1999 (01) Reporting Adverse Incidents Relating to Medical Devices. London: MDA Adverse Incident Centre.

Messina BAM (1994) Pulse oximetry: assuring accuracy. Journal of Post Anaesthesia Nursing 9(4), 228–231.

Moss F (1995) Risk management and quality of care. Quality in Health Care 4, 102–107.

NHS Executive (1994) Risk Management in the NHS. London: Department of Health.

NMC (2002) Guidelines for Records and Record-keeping. London: NMC.

Quine MA, Bell GD, McCloy RF, Charlton JE, Devlin HB, Hopkins A (1995) Prospective audit of upper gastrointestinal endoscopy in two regions of England: safety, staffing and sedation methods. Gut 36, 462–467.

Royal College of Nursing (1993) The Code of Practice for the Handling of Patients. London: RCN.

Royal College of Surgeons of England (1993) Guidelines for Sedation by Non-Anaesthetists. London: Department of External Affairs.

Sobala GM, Crabtree JE, Pentith JA, Rathbone BJ, Shallcross TM, Wyatt JI, Dixon MF, Heatley RV, Axon ATR (1991) Screening dyspepsia by serology to Helicobacter pylori. Lancet 338, 94–96.

Stafrace JG (1998) Assessment: the key to patient safety when undergoing an endoscopic procedure. Gastroenterology Nursing 21(3), 131–133.

Tingle J (1997) Clinical guidelines: legal and clinical risk management issues. British Journal of Nursing 6(11), 639–641.

UKCC (1989) Exercising Accountability. London: United Kingdom Central Council for Nursing, Midwifery and Health Visiting.

UKCC (1993) Standards for Records and Record Keeping. London: United Kingdom Central Council for Nursing, Midwifery and Health Visiting.

UKCC (1996) Guidelines for Professional Practice. London: United Kingdom Central Council for Nursing, Midwifery and Health Visiting.

Vanner SJ, MacDonald PH, Paterson WG, Prentice RSA, Da Costa LR, Beck IT (1990) A randomised prospective trial comparing oral sodium phosphate with standard polyethylene glycol-based lavage solution (Golytely) in the preparation of patients for colonoscopy. American Journal of Gastroenterology 85(4), 422–427.

Vincent C (1995) Clinical Risk Management. London: BMJ Publishing Group.

Wilson JH (1996) Integrated Care Management: the path to success? Oxford: Butterworth Heinemann.

CHAPTER 7

The legal position of nurses in clinical practice

MARIAN PEARSON

Introduction

The legal framework that governs nurses and nursing is one that is fairly complex in nature. Dimond (1995) describes the relationship between the law and nurses as arenas of accountability. Her diagrammatic representation of the professional at the centre surrounded by four main areas of accountability demonstrates that the nurse is accountable to patients, to the employer, to the profession and to the public. Respectively, the areas of law that govern these arenas are civil law, employment law, Nursing and Midwifery Council (NMC) Code of Professional Conduct (2002), and criminal law.

This chapter deals with each one of those arenas of accountability as separate issues. There is no doubt that they all link into one another, which demonstrates the complexity of the problems facing nurses in practice. The interlink between the law and the ethics of practice will thread throughout the various sections, as will nurses' accountability and responsibility.

External factors may vary over time, and will influence the position of nursing. Different opinions on the role of nursing within the provision of healthcare by successive governments are a major influence on the development or otherwise of the profession. Similar effects on individuals' rights as employees are generally in the hands of the government of the day. Some governments seek to improve the rights of the employee while other governments remove rights. Therefore, the reader should always seek up-to-date advice.

The two arenas that do remain reasonably static are in the area of civil and criminal law; however, expert advice and representation should also be sought when dealing with issues in these arenas.

Nurses in employment

Had this chapter been written ten years ago, this section would have began with a sentence which said, 'all nurses working in the National Health Service (NHS) are employed on Whitley Council Terms and conditions of service'. Today, however, nurses working in the NHS can be employed on such a variety of different terms and conditions of service that they are too numerous to list. Even more confusing is the way trusts pay their senior practitioners. Often the clinical grading structure does not reflect the roles of advanced practitioners and the only scheme for fair remuneration is the senior management pay spine. This is wholly unsatisfactory to those working in a clinical field, as it does not reflect their advanced skills and expertise. Nurses are advised to check their terms and conditions of service when moving posts, or taking up a new post with the same employer, and not assume that they are as previously enjoyed.

Hopefully this state of confusion may soon be remedied. The government has recognized the difficulties posed by the current systems and indeed the difficulties posed by the old 'Whitley' system. 'Agenda for Change' proposals are seeking to modernize the NHS pay scheme (DoH, 1999). The whole rationale, however, has to rely on a job evaluation system, which is currently being developed, capable of evaluating all jobs in the NHS. The central negotiating committee has ten agreed principles that will underpin any scheme.

Any proposal should meet the following principles:

- Assist ways of working which best deliver the range and quality of services required to meet the needs of patients.
- Achieve a quality workforce in the right numbers with the right skills and diversity.
- Improve recruitment and retention.
- Improve all aspects of equal opportunity, especially in career and training opportunities and working patterns that are not easily flexible to family commitments.
- Meet equal pay for work of equal value criteria.
- Be able to be implemented within the current management capacity.
- Apply to all staff employed in the NHS.

- Benefits for a changed system will outweigh the disadvantages.
- All aspects to be negotiated in the spirit of social partnership.
- Consistent with the National Human Resource Strategy.

The new scheme should be up and running by April 2003. We currently await more definitive proposals.

What does, however, remain static is the relationship between the employer and the employee. The employee carries out specific duties for the employer for a specified remuneration package. It is important that this relationship occurs in this manner, as there are a number of statute laws that rely on this relationship. Young (1995) confirms that the employer and employees have both rights and duties, which is an important fact that needs to be recognized.

The employees' rights are enshrined within the Employment Protection (Consolidation) Act 1978. There have been further significant pieces of legislation since 1974 that impinge on the aforementioned Act, but it still remains the basis by which the rights of the employee can be enforced. For example, an improvement to the employees' rights occurred following the implementation of the Trade Union and Employment Rights Act 1993. This Act removed the qualifying period for all claims of breaches of statutory rights, i.e. pregnancy and maternity leave; the provision of written terms and conditions of service.

An employee can bring about a claim for unfair dismissal should the employer act unreasonably. The employee must have been employed by the employer for one year in order to qualify to bring about a claim for unfair dismissal. Until very recently the qualifying period was two years of continuous service. This feature of employees' rights changes regularly and individuals should always seek advice regarding the current position.

As employees have rights, so do employers. We have to recognize that we live in a changing world, and within healthcare the pace of change remains as rapid as ever. Managers are often in the position of reorganizing and changing services to meet the needs of patients. Nursing posts may alter as a result, and all staff need to be supported through the uncertainties that ensue. It is often difficult for staff working in a department to have knowledge of the wider picture of the provision of healthcare in their locality. The introduction of Primary Care Trusts (PCTs) will inevitably refocus the purchasing of services that currently sit within the acute sector.

For example, a PCT may decide as a priority that it would provide greater benefit to the health of more patients by purchasing health promotion specialist advice. As a consequence there will be less money for routine work and, as such, the members of staff delivering that service will have fewer customers. Assessing the need to continue to provide this service must then be the responsibility of the acute trust. It is without doubt that in these circumstances services would have to change. The impact of this change on nurses, doctors and other health professionals would mean massive changes in their work. Retraining for new ways of working will be a major consideration in the health service over the coming years.

Health and safety

Employees, as previously discussed, have duties under their contract of employment. For example, the contract of employment expects that they will abide by the rules set out in policies and procedures by their employer. Failure to do so may bring about a dismissal that is fair. The Health and Safety at Work Act 1974 also gives the employee a duty, which is fundamental to their function at work. The expectation of the Act is that the employer has a duty to provide a safe working environment, but the duty of the employee is to ensure that:

- they maintain a safe working environment for themselves and others
- they utilize any equipment provided by the employer which has been deemed necessary in the discharge of their duties.

For example: patient A is assessed on admission. The patient is immobile and requires lifting and handling to the toilet and bathroom. The patient weighs 15 stone. The trained assessor confirms that the patient should be moved by mechanical hoist and instructions are documented in the patient's records. In this situation, the employer has a duty to the patient (duty of care) and the staff (Health and Safety at Work Act) to provide the equipment necessary. The staff caring for that patient have the duty to use the equipment provided in the manner that has been advised.

The influence of European legislation on our health and safety, and indeed employment, rights is now significant. Legislation, regulations and directives all influence the working environment. The Working Time Directive is a very complex piece of legislation. It has been introduced to combat the ill-health effects of work, particularly shift work. It controls the amount of time that individuals need to rest between shifts. The ultimate aim is to produce a healthier workforce, by ensuring that workers rest, and long shifts are shortened.

Nurses and the Nursing and Midwifery Council

A nurse is a registered professional and as such is placed on the roll by the NMC. The Nursing and Midwifery Coucil took over from the UKCC in April 2002. A review of the Nurses, Midwives and Health Visitors Act 1979 led to the inception of the NMC. New legislation was required to replace the existing regulatory structure with one that is more modern and responsive.

The NMC has 24–27 members as a central strategic body, with equal representation of elected nurses and midwives from each UK country. The Council has a professional majority with one third of the representatives being lay members.

The functions of the NMC are fundamental to the development of nurses and nursing practice. It has a much stronger emphasis than its predecessor on the protection of the public. While preparation for practice is an important element supporting the development of nurses and nursing practice, the previous work done by the UKCC through education boards will not continue in the same way.

The NMC Code of Conduct (2002) reminds us that nurses are accountable for their own actions. The *Oxford English Dictionary* definition for accountable is 'responsible: required to account for one's actions'. Nurses must be aware of current practice and always act in the best interests of patients. As previously discussed, it is insufficient to carry out instructions from other professional groups without understanding the issues involved. It is the responsibility of the nurse to check the patient's understanding of the situation. The legal perspective of accountability will be discussed in greater detail under 'civil liability'.

Professional Conduct Committee

One of the fundamental functions of the NMC is to regulate practitioners, thereby improving their professional standards and conduct. Any member of the general public can report a registered nurse to the NMC. There is a duty on the NMC to investigate all matters that are reported to them.

The NMC has the power to suspend a practitioner immediately from practice if the nature of the complaint is so serious as to cause concern for the public, or if it is deemed to be in the best interest of the practitioner.

Once it is established that there is a case to answer, the matter is referred to the Professional Conduct Committee. This committee must determine whether or not the practitioner is guilty of misconduct. Three courses of action are then available to it:

- to issue a caution as to future conduct;
- with a view to removal of the practitioner's name from the register;
- it may consider a practitioner's fitness to practise, whereupon the Health Committee would deal with the matter from there on.

In recent times, the continuum of care of patients has changed significantly. At one time nurses were involved only in nursing tasks and medical staff were involved in most invasive procedures. Today, the nurse is involved in a wide variety of clinical procedures, which used to be the sole domain of the doctor. Significant debate within the profession has ensued. The vision for the future of the nursing profession, as outlined in the nursing strategy *Making a Difference* (NHSE, 1999), gives professionals and managers clear indications that the tide is not likely to change. The government document gives us a clear indication that they will enable and encourage the nursing profession to extend its role and responsibilities in the quest of improving patient care and outcomes.

What duties can be properly delegated to a nurse? In many circumstances the changes have been incremental and have often reflected changes in medical practice. For example, coronary care units were set up in the 1970s purely for the swift treatment of patients who might suffer a cardiac arrest following a myocardial infarction. Nurses were on duty 24 hours a day because it was recognized that these incidents could occur at any time and known that delay in providing treatment decreases the patient's life expectancy. Nurses were trained to take on a role that was clinically more involved than their basic training. Tasks such as intubation, intravenous (IV) infusion, administration of drugs via agreed protocols and defibrillation were added to their credentials. The profession has moved on into many different areas of patient care since then.

The UKCC Scope of Professional Practice (1992) indicates that nursing practice should be directed by patient need and not, as has been attempted in recent times, a shortage of medical staff. However, they do advise that practitioners exercise caution, in that any developments in nursing should not compromise existing aspects of care.

Nurse prescribing

Nurses have been involved in the prescription of medication for many years. Midwives in particular have prescribed drugs for the use of patients during childbirth. HSC 1998/051 (NHSE, 1998) advised health authorities, following a review, about the supply and administration of medicines under group protocols.

The development of nurse prescribing has met many difficulties, particularly in the legislative field. Guidelines for implementation of protocols are now available within most community trusts. In some instances, nurses have led the project team, which consists of medical and pharmaceutical staff, in working up these guidelines. Further advice is available from the Royal Colleges of Nursing and Medicine.

Patient Group Direction (PGD) arrangements, however, do not fall entirely within the Medicines Act. The NMC and the RCN agree that a safe and properly thought out protocol is a safe and effective way of meeting patients' needs. The legal debate continues to cause concern to practitioners. The Crown Review set up a number of criteria that should be met when agreeing protocols.

• Patients should receive medication on an individual basis in certain limited situations.
• The law should be clarified to encompass all health professionals and include those (nurses) who supply or administer medicines.
• Protocols should take account of patient choice and convenience.
• PGD protocols should not normally be used in the case of drugs under intensive monitoring and subject to special adverse reaction; unlicensed medicines; medicines being used in clinical trials.

The benefit to patients regarding the implementation of the nurse prescribing scheme is yet to be assessed.

Continuing professional development

As part of its initial brief, the UKCC was charged with the duty to improve standards of patient care and the development of the profession. We have previously discussed a number of ways in which it carried out this function. The UKCC, following extensive consultation with the profession, agreed a framework for qualified staff to develop after their initial training in order to re-register. This is now up and running and nurses are expected to provide evidence of study and development of their practice as a result of this study. Nurses who have been out of practice for more than five years are expected to undertake a return-to-practice programme. It is expected that the NMC will develop this work further.

Higher level of practice

In response to the developments in nursing care that have been ongoing for many years, the UKCC consulted with its members regarding a proposed regulatory framework for nurses, midwives and health visitors who are working at a higher level of practice.

> Practitioners working at a higher level act as leaders for change with the public, patients and clients. They cross professional and agency boundaries to achieve this. They network, locally, regionally and nationally, and recognise the ethical, legal and professional constraints on practice. They assess and manage risk. Those working at a higher level have aspects of education, research and management included within their role but the main focus, purpose and impact of their work are patients, clients or communities
>
> (UKCC, 1999).

It is expected that the assessment process will focus on practice. Practitioners will be asked to present evidence of their achievements in the form of a portfolio. The portfolio will be scrutinized to confirm that the necessary evidence is available. Practitioners will then be visited at their workplace to verify the evidence and provide contextual information for assessment by a panel. The panel will then meet and discuss its contents with the practitioner. Guidance for candidates is available from the NMC.

This is a welcome development for many nurses. The new framework will provide a formal recognition for the developments they have undertaken. However, a change of legislation will be required to enable the registration of such individuals.

Civil liability

Nursing, as we discussed in the previous section, is a self-regulating profession. It does this through the powers of the NMC. That does not make the nurse immune from other liabilities.

There is an increasing number of professionals who are called to account for their actions, not only in their own professional courts but also within the civil and criminal courts.

Any member of the public in the UK is entitled to seek legal advice to sue a professional for a negligent act. Often actions such as these are directed towards the employer, who carries vicarious liability, but more frequently now actions are directed at individuals. Most professionals carry professional indemnity insurance, which supports them and covers any costs, including legal and damages, in the event they are sued. Those professionals who practise without such insurance have little regard for their patients who may be damaged as a result of the professional's actions and have no opportunity to seek compensation.

The lengthy process involved in such action can often deter individuals. Negligence has to be demonstrated by them in order to be successful. There are three elements when considering a negligence action, all of which have to be proven.

- The patient has to demonstrate that the defendant owes a duty of care to him or her.
- The patient has to prove that there is a breach in the standard of the duty of care.
- This breach must have caused damage.

There are other schemes available in other countries. In New Zealand, a no-fault compensation scheme exists. In this type of scheme the patient who has been damaged does not have to prove who is negligent. They must, however, prove that the damage would not reasonably occur under normal circumstances. This procedure is beneficial to all and in particular to the patients, who are not as well supported financially as the larger organizations to progress through long legal battles.

What is not in question, however, is the standard of care that is required. All courts use the Bolam test – 'the standard of the ordinary skilled man exercising and professing to have that special skill' – to determine negligence. Lee (1995) argues that the objectivity of the standard is crucial. He observes that the law will not consider the human failings in determining a breach of the duty of care. People, health professionals included, have different ways in which they perform their jobs. The standard that will be used will be that of a nurse with similar qualifications and experience. For example, a clinical nurse specialist is involved in an incident whereby a patient dies as a result of a feeding tube being inserted into the lungs and not the stomach. The court would apply the Bolam test and would not use the newly qualified staff nurse as the control group. They would seek evidence from similarly qualified nurses as to the skills expected of this group of specialists.

Vicarious liability

'Employers are liable for any negligent acts committed by their employees under the doctrine of "vicarious liability"'(Montgomery, 1995). A trust has a duty to provide healthcare services to a local population. It discharges its duty of care to its employees who deliver the service to the population. In vicarious liability, the employer will be held responsible for the actions of the staff – even those who are negligent. However, there is an increasing trend by trusts to attempt to recover some of the monies paid to patients in damages claims by claiming from medical and nursing indemnity insurance schemes.

Indemnity insurance schemes are usually provided via membership of organizations such as the RCN. Private indemnity insurance can also be sought, but the cost is usually prohibitive. An indemnity insurance scheme is similar to car insurance in that if you have a cover note that commences at 12 noon, and you have an accident at 11.45am, then the insurance will not be valid. Similarly, if your membership of an organization has ceased the insurance will not cover any mistakes that you make while caring for patients during that time. Rules of the scheme are available from the organization that provides the scheme. It is essential that nurses carry indemnity insurance, and some employers within the private healthcare sector insist on membership of an organization as a prerequisite to employment.

Informed consent

Patients have a right under common law to give or withhold consent prior to treatment. Employers will have debated the issues and agreed policies with all groups of staff who are directly involved in gaining consent from patients. If a patient is touched without consent, they will have the right of action in the civil courts of suing either the practitioner or the employer.

The law requires that before treatment is given, consent is obtained from the patient. Without consent, the nurse is failing in her responsibilities to the patient and to the employer, which will ultimately result in attendance in civil or criminal court. This duty falls to the nurse more readily than any other group of professionals in two ways. First, the nurse may be carrying out procedures under the instruction of medical staff. In this instance it is the nurse's responsibility to ensure that the patient wishes to comply with the procedure. Second, where the doctor has gained consent, the nurse may be aware that the patient has not understood the full extent of the discussions. The nurse is responsible to the patient and to her employer to give advice and clarification to the patient if there is any misunderstanding about the procedure, and should inform the medical staff of this problem.

The scenarios above are examples of express consent, where a patient has signed a document giving consent to a procedure. There are millions of examples every day of patient interaction where a nurse or doctor interfaces with patients and carries out invasive procedures where a signed document is not used. These are examples of implied consent, for example, in the GP surgery, where significant numbers of patients come through the system on a daily basis. The patient sees the doctor, who advises that a blood test is required to reach a diagnosis and provide effective treatment. The patient then visits the nurse for the blood test, but unbeknown to the patient, one of the tests to be carried out is for HIV. The implications for the patient, in this scenario, are considerable. It may inhibit his or her ability to obtain insurance and employment. Nurses who collaborate in this procedure in these circumstances could be reported to the NMC for misconduct. The ethical considerations here of course may be very different. It may be argued that, in some circumstances, it is in the best interests of the patient to ascertain the information. UKCC (1994) guidelines will allow unconsented testing only in 'rare and exceptional circumstances'.

Gaining the patient's consent will generally be seen as a defence against any action for trespass or assault. The patient is entitled to receive sufficient information that he or she is able to understand. Gaining consent in certain circumstances may not be enough to defend a negligence action, the details of which have been discussed earlier in this chapter. A patient may not understand the consequences of the treatment. Health professionals need to ensure that they take all reasonable steps to be certain that the patient understands what is to happen and the effects of the treatment. A locally agreed policy is always the best way forward, provided that it sits within Department of Health guidelines HC (90) 22. There are a number of specialist groups that have formulated policies and guidelines specific to the client group and the procedures that may be used. The British Society of Gastroenterology guidelines for informed consent for endoscopic procedures (BSG, 1999) deal with the overall issues around consent and more directly with the thorny issues that are specific to this group of patients.

How much do we tell the patient? This must also be of concern to healthcare professionals. If staff fail to inform the patient of the risks of complication involved with the procedure and that patient subsequently suffers one of the complications, he or she may decide to seek a negligence claim. In the case of *Sidaway* v *Board of Governors of Bethlem Royal Hospital* (1985), the patient underwent surgery for recurrent neck pain. There was an underlying risk, albeit small, of injury to the spinal column. The patient was left severely disabled after the operation. The case of negligence eventually failed, despite the fact that the surgeon had informed the patient of certain risks but had not informed her of this particular risk.

The House of Lords accepted that the surgeon had acted as a similar qualified doctor would have acted at the time. It is therefore incumbent on healthcare professionals to be aware of recent developments in practice and to act within guidelines offered by professional bodies. Best practice must be to make the patient aware of all risks and benefits that may occur and allow him or her to decide on the approach that should be taken.

Criminal liability

Nurses can find themselves subjected to criminal proceedings. This may happen in a variety of ways and can occur at work as well as outside of work. There are a number of factors to consider at this point.

- Nurses are civilians in the community. They can be charged and found guilty of offences from their civilian life, for example a drunk-driving offence. This conviction may have implications in their working life. Speaking to various groups of nurses it appears that this issue is a little contentious. Some nurses believe that minor convictions should not impact on their position at work or indeed be of interest to the NMC. Others take a different view in that the privilege that is afforded to a nurse by patients should not be harmed in any way. Employers and the NMC do, however, have a view. The Code of Professional Conduct (NMC, 2002) offers the rules by which nurses should conduct themselves both in work and outside of work.
- Nurses are exempt from the Rehabilitation of Offenders Act 1974. They must inform their employer of any previous criminal offence prior to employment, and any conviction that occurs while in employment. Failure to do so may lead the employer to believe that the 'trust' (implied in the contract of employment) between the two parties has irrevocably broken down. This would give the employer reasonable grounds on which to dismiss.
- Nurses who are convicted of a criminal offence will be reported through the courts to the NMC. Depending on the offence, the NMC may take a view that the matter should be dealt with by the Professional Conduct Committee.

- There are a number of cases where healthcare professionals have committed criminal acts within their working environment. Nurses have been found guilty of crimes such as theft of drugs and assault through to manslaughter and murder. Again, in these circumstances, the NMC would take a view as to the practitioner's fitness to remain on the Register, as well as the sentence that would be imposed on the individual by the criminal courts.

Record keeping

In this chapter we have discussed a variety of ways in which nurses can become involved in legal situations, i.e. in a civil court, NMC court, criminal court or employment tribunal. Even within an internal setting, nurses may have to rely on their entries in patient records, sometimes many years after the event.

The standard of legal care that is required by law is to act as an ordinary skilled nurse would have acted in the circumstances of the case. Patient records can be produced as evidence in a court of law. There will be local protocols for record keeping and these should be adhered to. The NMC offers guidance to nurses in this regard. The Standards for Records and Record Keeping (UKCC, 1993) offers the following points in guidance. Records should provide:

- comprehensive picture of care
- pertinent information
- evidence of the duty of care
- continued care/discharge arrangements
- problems that deviate from the norm
- identification of the entrant.

The UKCC also offers specific guidance on patient-held records, patients' access to records, shared records and computer-held records, which will be updated by the NMC in the near future.

Statement writing

Nurses are often asked to write a statement regarding an incident that has occurred. This is often the time when the nurse has to return to the written record of care to remind herself of the patient and the circumstances in which she cared for him or her. Sometimes this can be requested several years after an event and the only reliable evidence is the nursing notes. If practitioners have stayed within the guidelines as previously discussed, then the statement will be easier to produce.

Whatever the reason for requesting a statement, be it a patient care incident, an accident or a workplace incident, the following principles apply:

- The date and time of the incident should be made clear on the first and all subsequent pages.
- You should state your name, position, grade and location.
- You should name all persons involved.
- You should give a full description of the event leading up to and following the event, provided that it is relevant.
- You should include any supporting evidence.
- The document should be signed with the date and time that it was completed.
- Keep a copy for yourself. Remember that litigation can take up to seven years from the date of the incident.

Ethics

While various sections of this chapter have already touched on the notion of ethics, it is valuable to discuss the relationship between ethical values and the legal framework. The two notions often get confused.

Beauchamp and Childress (1989) established four principles, which have been widely used in healthcare:

- respect autonomy
- harming
- where possible, benefit
- consider the interests of all those affected.

Nursing values and the framework in which nurses' work can sometimes bring them into conflict with other health professionals and their employer. Allocation of resources can often cause conflict between these groups. For example, a nurse assesses a patient with a stoma, who has previously had prescribed treatment within the PGD. The nurse assesses that the dressing used is not compatible with the patient's needs. To change the dressing would cause less discomfort to the patient and prevent further complications that would protract the course of the illness.

Simultaneously the trust issues instructions to staff to remain within the protocol as the trust has a severe overspend. The dilemma for the nurse in these circumstances is one that nurses face every day. The patient's needs are clear, as are the employer's, but the two do not match and the nurse is torn between them – neither can be ignored. Advice from a senior manager should be sought in these circumstances.

A nurse's employment may be placed in jeopardy should she fail to comply with the request from the trust. Similarly, should the patient bring about a negligence action, the nurse would have to account for her actions and provide supporting evidence to defend the decision made.

Conclusion

This chapter has considered the areas in which nurses are accountable and how they all interlink with one another. There are no easy answers to many of the questions that may be posed by practitioners. The fundamental perspective remains that nurses are responsible for their practice and cannot hide behind other professional groups to protect them.

Nurses can now follow an exciting path, developing into areas that have previously been the domain of other healthcare professionals, yet maintaining the core skills required to preserve the nurse–patient relationship. Nursing is the profession that is best placed to develop in this way, with the patient at the core.

The legal framework in which nurses work has changed, and will continue to change, to allow this development. As nurses' skills move away from the more traditional role to one that is more innovative, their position within the law also changes.

References

Beauchamp TL, Childress JF (1989) Principles of Biomedical Ethics. New York: Oxford University Press.

British Society of Gastroenterology (1999) Guidelines for Informed Consent for Endoscopic Procedures. http://www.bsg.org.uk

Department of Health Health service management patient consent to examination or treatment. HC (90) 22.

Department of Health (1999) Agenda for change. London: HMSO.

Dimond BC (1995) Legal Aspects of Nursing, 2nd edn. London: Prentice Hall

Lee R (1995) In: Tingle J, Cribb A (eds) Nursing Law and Ethics. Oxford: Blackwell Science.

Montgomery J (1995) In: Tingle J, Cribb A (eds) Nursing Law and Ethics. Blackwell Science.

NHS Executive (1998) The Review of Prescribing, Supply and Administration of Medicines. HSC 1998/051. London: HMSO.

NHS Executive (1999) Making a Difference. London: HMSO.

NMC (2002) Code of Professional Conduct. London: NMC.

UKCC (1992) Scope of Professional Practice. London: UKCC.

UKCC (1993) Standards for Records and Record Keeping. London: UKCC.

UKCC (1994) Aids and HIV Infection; the council's position statement. London: UKCC.

UKCC (1999) A Higher Level of Practice Pilot. London: UKCC.

Young A (1995) In: Tingle J, Cribb A (eds) Nursing Law and Ethics. Blackwell Science.

CHAPTER 8

Health-promoting practice

JULIE DICKINSON and STELLA JONES-DEVITT

Introduction

Health promotion theory and practice is a broad area of study. This chapter includes an exploration of patient-centred practice, collaborative working, health promotion as a catalyst for change and the use of evidence-based practice. Each section is supplemented by exercises for the reader to try; these help to relate the theory to practice. The final section provides a framework for developing and implementing a practice development plan around the main themes discussed. In addition, the reader is directed towards some key sources that help to explore in further depth the themes outlined.

Patient-centred practice

Patient-centred practice has become a common healthcare term in recent times. However, its use in both theory and practice seems to suggest that it is interpreted and implemented differently, depending on the writer or practitioner. This section discusses the differing views of health and their importance, and explores the theory and practice of patient-led approaches in health-promoting practice.

Establishing a patient's view of the constituents of health (or healthy behaviour) is vitally important if any subsequent action is to be patient-centred. In looking at various concepts of health, Ewles and Simnett (1999) refer to it holistically as incorporating physical, mental, emotional, social, spiritual and societal health. An example of this holistic concept related to gastroenterology is discussed by Ross (1998), who suggests that in relation to constipation, emotional, psychological, environmental and dietary (physical) factors all need to be taken into account when promoting patient health.

Another popular way to explore health is to categorize various factors under three main models: medical, salutogenic and social. The medical model of health tends to define health in relation to illness. Examples of this approach include health assessments based on disease or lifestyle issues (McBride, 1995), evaluating the outcome of exercise programmes for patients with inflammatory bowel disease (Ball, 1998) and using patient education videos (Abbott, 1998). The medical model is characterized by power relationships between professional and patient, with the latter being seen as a passive recipient of expert knowledge and intervention (Jones, 1997). Interestingly, some professionals view this model as patient-centred, as although the needs are defined by the professional, subsequent action is for the patient's benefit (Campbell, 1998).

The salutogenic model of health can be interpreted as more patient-centred. This model, developed by Antonovsky (1993), suggests that the normal 'lived experience' for most people is one of disorder, and that health and disease oscillate within this haphazardness.

Fundamentally, the salutogenic model defines health as the ability to cope with life and all its complexities. Managing depends not only on personal resources, but also on relationships, social support and supportive environments (Antonovsky, 1993). Research into health needs of patients with irritable bowel disease found that the ability to cope with the condition was an important factor in promoting their health and overall quality of life (Smolen and Topp, 1997).

The final model of health to be discussed is the social model, which is related strongly to contemporary thinking in health promotion (Jones, 1997). This model considers multicausal theories for health status, suggesting that health is influenced by political, economic, social, psychological and cultural aspects, as well as biological factors. It centres on starting with the client's needs, which corresponds well to a patient-centred ethos. Jones (1997) notes that its guiding principles concern commitment to empowerment, local participation, equity in health, accountability and co-operation with other agencies. Robinson and Hill (1998) also suggest that the needs of the patient must be considered in the broadest possible context. This is discussed in relation to the health-promoting nurse role.

Exercise

- Consider your view of health in your professional setting, which model of health does it relate to the most?

• Consider your patients' views of health and to which model(s) they relate.

Patient-centred practice is presented as one of the core principles of health-promoting practice, demonstrated globally by the World Health Organization's targets for *Health For All* (WHO, 1985) and nationally in the UK government's recent White Paper *Saving Lives: our healthier nation* (DoH, 1999b). It is also considered in various ways by the many different models and definitions of health promotion.

When exploring the theory and practice of health promotion, many different ways of practising emerge. Ewles and Simnett (1999), in discussing approaches to health promotion, state that there is no one right approach and it is dependent on our 'own professional code of conduct (if there is one), our own carefully considered values and our own assessment of our client's needs' (Ewles and Simnett, 1999, p41). Approaches that could be viewed as more patient-centred include: client-centred, educational and societal change approaches. The client-centred approach concerns treating clients as equals who then have the right to set any agendas. This involves working with the clients on their own terms, where solely the client defines both the content and approach. The educational approach could be seen to be patient-centred as it purportedly gives the client information, which they then rationalize independently of the health professional. However, it is still the health promoter, rather than the patient, who takes responsibility for the choice of topic and content. The societal change approach is concerned with altering the physical and social environment in order to enable 'healthier lifestyle' choices. This could be viewed as either patient-centred or expert-led, depending on who sets the agendas. Examples of expert-led health promotion include the implementation of a no-smoking policy in a hospital, government laws on wearing seatbelts and under-age drinking. Examples of patient-centred perspectives include: local community groups campaigning for a school crossing and a patients' council deciding on health-related hospital policies such as visiting times.

The final two approaches defined by Ewles and Simnett (1999) are medical and behaviour change, which are concerned with patient compliance, in which health is defined solely by the health promoter. These approaches correspond to the medical view of health discussed earlier, where disease prevention and early detection are encouraged, along with lifestyle behaviour change (Jones, 1997).

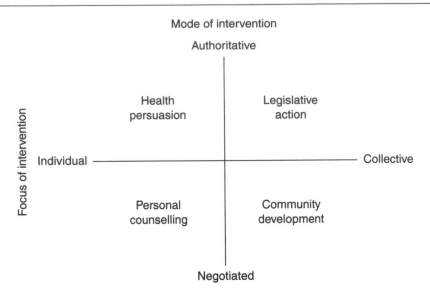

Figure 8.1 Approaches to health promotion. (Source: Beattie, 1991).

Another way of exploring health promotion is through its various models. Beattie (1991) clearly separates patient-centred approaches to health promotion. His model (Figure 8.1) refers to a mode of intervention, which is either authoritative (expert-led) or negotiated (patient-centred).

By presenting his model in this way, Beattie concentrates more on exploring and analysing the values that govern practice (Jones and Naidoo, 1997) rather than just describing practice, as in Ewles and Simnett's (1999) model. His quadrant of health persuasion fits well with Ewles and Simnett's medical and behaviour change approaches; while personal counselling corresponds to the client-centred approach. Jones and Naidoo (1997) suggest that the social change approach of Ewles and Simnett indicates a commitment which relates to Beattie's community development quadrant; however, if the former approach is more expert-led, then this could have more in common with legislative action. Caplan and Holland (1990) also support the view that health promotion theory should look further than just describing practice. They state that the health promoter's view of society (reflecting the need to make radical change or to conform to existing social regulations) will affect their practice. In addition (and of particular importance to patient-centred care) is whether the health promoter believes that knowledge is either objectified, and therefore defined by experts; or subjective, and grounded in human experience.

Exercise

Consider your practice in relation to both Ewles and Simnett's (1999) approaches to health promotion and Beattie's (1991) model.

• Where does your practice sit at present?
• How could you change your practice to make it more patient-centred?

As stated earlier, patient-centred practice is problematic to define, yet one ideal germane to all attempts at a definition concerns the need to actively empower patients (Campbell, 1998; Tones et al., 1990). Empowerment of communities and individuals has been a fundamental aim of health promotion since the Ottawa Charter (WHO, 1986). Here, empowerment is seen as the mechanism where individuals, organizations and communities are enabled to gain mastery over their lives, thereby having control to improve their health (WHO, 1986). Tones et al. (1990) advocate the importance of this approach in health promotion, seeing that its effective implementation comes through education. In addition, Ewles and Simnett's (1999) client-centred approach and Beattie's (1991) negotiated quadrants all reflect the importance of empowerment notions in health promotion.

One of the key issues regarding implementation of empowerment processes concerns the idea that nurses are generally a disempowered professional body, which then makes it difficult to empower patients (Latter, 1998; Wilson-Barnett and Latter, 1993). If this is the case, then consideration has to be made to provide structures which ensure that nurses have more control over their own practice, prior to attempting the empowerment of patients. Other issues include whether the patients actually desire empowerment (Campbell, 1998; Latter, 1998). Empowerment notions and patient-centredness become problematic if patients choose to pass over autonomy to the experts (Woodward, 1998; Campbell, 1998). Wider issues include the need to consider how empowering society is for patients beyond the hospital setting (Latter, 1998) and patients' ability to sustain being empowered in the context of their own community (Campbell, 1998).

In conclusion, when exploring a more patient-centred approach to health promotion, it is useful to reflect on the motivation behind such approaches, especially if, as suggested by Ewles and Simnett (1999), there is no right approach. One motivation is its association with obtaining successful changes of behaviour. Saddler (1999) discusses the importance of considering the patient's needs in her article on education for the gastroenterology patient. She notes that a patient is more likely to learn and act on such learning if their needs are seen to be taken into account. The motivation underlying this type of patient-centred practice can often be interpreted as tokenistic (Meyer, 1993). These differing views are discussed in more detail in later sections.

Although obtaining a successful outcome is as important in health promotion as in other areas of healthcare practice, it could be argued that the true essence of patient-centred care should be concerned principally with patients' rights. Fundamentally, this relates to autonomy and self-determination regarding individuals' 'lived experience'. A provocative piece of analysis by Maynard (1995) entitled 'Is killing people wrong?' argues that policies that restrict people's rights to smoke or drink could be seen as morally wrong, as they constrain freedom and are based on society's values. If a health professional suggests, promotes or encourages a course of action for a patient, which is based on the professional's own values and judgement, this could also be seen as restricting freedom and influencing choice. Woodward (1998) sees possible tensions between beneficence and autonomy where a nurse sees a patient's decision as being harmful. If patient-centred care is about supporting the wishes of the patient, then respecting autonomy and patients' rights to determine their own lives (including medically defined 'damaging' behaviour) could be seen as doing more good and preventing less harm.

Collaborative working

Collaborative practice in health promotion, as in all forms of healthcare practice, operates in many different ways. This section explores the theory and practice from an inter-agency and inter-professional perspective, while examining levels of participation and its implementation on a team and managerial basis.

In defining collaboration from a nursing perspective, the Joint Committee of Professional Nursing, Midwifery and Health Visitor Associations in England (1997) sees it as a way of providing a seamless service across professional and agency boundaries, with all partners contributing to service delivery decisions and future developments. However, Leathard (1997) explores the debate further by discussing a dictionary definition, which implies a form of co-operation with the enemy, yet moving towards working together. The common element underpinning both perspectives concerns the potential for collaboration. However, Leathard (1997) also demonstrates potential problems of its implementation in practice.

There is no question that collaborative practice is supported from a policy perspective. Examples of this from a health promotion perspective include:

- the government White Paper *Saving Lives: our healthier nation* (DoH, 1999b)
- more focused policies like *Smoking Kills* (DoH, 1998b) and the *Acheson Report on Inequalities in Health* (DoH, 1998a)
- nursing policies such as *Making a Difference* (DoH, 1999a) and the UKCC *Code of Professional Conduct* (UKCC, 1992).

All stress the importance of collaboration with professionals and clients in primary and secondary care. Collaborative working is also a key tenet of *The New NHS: modern, dependable* (DoH, 1997) – a policy that sets the framework for existing and future healthcare practice. Inter-agency collaboration is seen as essential for successful health-promoting practice: 'If health promotion policies are to improve the nation's health, inter-agency collaboration is essential' (Skinner, 1995, p193).

Encouraging agencies to work together to improve the health of the population seems the obvious approach when the factors that contribute to ill health are so diverse. As listed above, government policies are promoting inter-agency work, yet consideration needs to be given as to how this can be implemented in practice. Developing inter-agency working even between elements of the NHS could be seen as problematic, as this has introduced changes to established ways of working.

The development of the internal market started with the Griffiths Report (1983) resulting in the White Paper *Working for Patients* (DoH, 1989). This created a culture of competing for resources, rather than encouraging collaboration (Ham, 1999). It could also be argued that inter-agency working resulting in collaboration is not enough: to truly co-operate, trans-disciplinary working needs to exist, in which a new set of shared values and ways of working are considered from the outset. This approach (as discussed by Ovretveit, 1993) should result in more equitable working relationships between agencies. The issues for inter-agency collaboration are also reflected in inter-professional and inter-disciplinary working. Albrecht et al. (1998) support Ovretveit (1993) in citing the importance of trans-disciplinary working utilizing a common conceptual framework. However, obtaining a common cross-disciplinary culture can be threatening to some professional groups. Nursing can be seen to be very territorial (Gottlieb and Gottlieb, 1998), therefore presenting barriers to other professionals, even including other groups of nurses (Pike, 1995).

Exercise

- List all the individuals and agencies you collaborate with. Reflect on how this collaboration works in practice.
- In particular, consider whether you have agreed ways of carrying out health-promoting practice.

Collaboration, it could be argued, should also include patients and carers. As indicated in earlier sections, if patient-centred practice is the desired goal, then the patient must surely be seen as an equal partner in their care. This ideal is clearly supported theoretically by the policies mentioned earlier. Indeed, *Making a Difference* (DoH, 1999a) states this clearly as a key practice objective. Practitioners may wish to ponder on whether this reflects their own practice. Leathard (1997) suggests that the patient not only needs equal power in relation to others, but that consideration needs to be given concerning whether collaborating with other agencies will provide tangible benefits. Fundamental issues to consider include confidentiality and impact on continuity of care. In terms of encouraging successful collaboration, Sidell (1997) suggests that group and teamwork theories need to be explored alongside organizational and management models, which include overt patient involvement.

Successful teamworking is a skill that needs to be practised like any other. Practical considerations include:

- identifying all the team members
- establishing a common purpose
- understanding the importance of recognizing relevant expertise
- building a knowledge of each other's roles.

In continuing the teamwork, there must be continued support, trust and continuity (Ewles and Simnett, 1999). Forster (1995) supports the continued development of teamwork to ensure collaborative practice. She notes that benefits include both improved standards of care and increased job satisfaction, achieved through mutual support.

From a management perspective, collaborative practice can be even more problematic, with conflict developing between preserving specific organizational interests and constructing policies that direct agencies to work together for a common good (Naidoo and Wills, 1998). Practical solutions again tend to come back to the importance of shared goals and value systems, with a commitment to embracing change and further inter-agency development.

Exercise

- Do you operate as a member of any work-based team?
- Work through Ewles and Simnett's (1999) considerations for effective teamwork. Are they all achieved?

It appears that collaborative practice is an ideal that is supported presently both in theory and in directions for future practice. Its implementation may be harder to achieve, due to established cultures between and within organizations. As discussed earlier, if its development is sustained in practice then this may result in considerable improvement for health enhancement strategies.

Health promotion as a catalyst for change

This section looks at some of the strategies that can be used when managing change in health promotion environments. It also considers how both theory and reflective practice processes can contribute to managing change more effectively, and explores the need to ground change processes in a wider political context.

Social relations and institutions are exposed to escalating change processes in a fast-moving global environment. Health promotion environments need to respond quickly if they are to remain conducive to enhancing health. In order to flourish within a constantly evolving world, both individuals and organizations need to accept that certain principles apply (Handy, 1991). Like risk, change is neither 'good' nor 'bad'; it just *is*. Change is always subject to differing perceptions and 'truths' dependent on the agendas of the agents involved; change doesn't stop – social structures may have periods of overall relative stability, yet still experience change dynamics at microcosmic and interactive levels on a daily basis. Even when no obvious new output emerges, the process of change still ensures that the new situation is different from previous states. The health-promoting practitioner needs to be able to make sense of these complex processes and ground them within their own experience and working context (Katz and Peberdy, 1997).

Exercise

- How much change have you experienced in your professional role over the past three years?
- How much of that change do you perceive to be positive?

Developing an understanding of change at an individual level and then interpreting organizational change in relation to individual functioning is an essential part of any sense-making toolkit. At an individual level, the practitioner needs to employ active learning strategies in line with the move towards more reflexive approaches in nursing. Schon (1983) describes the process of learning as a way of dealing with change. He suggests there is an exchange between theory and practice when practitioners reflect effectively. Consider the following sequence:

1   The practitioner realizes that there is an unsatisfactory situation in their work context and ponders whether the theory which underlies the practice is appropriate.
2   The practitioner introduces a new practice approach which they hope will produce more satisfactory outcomes.
3   The resulting outcomes of the new approach are evaluated against the existing ones. If the move has failed to produce the results intended, then the practitioner revisits the theory that led to false expectations (Schon calls this a 'theory response to error').

In this process, the practitioner surfaces the underlying theory, criticizes it, rebuilds it, then tests the new theory by inventing a new move in their practice approach. However, if the outcomes of the new approach have been successful in terms of improved outcomes, then the new move is adopted and the existing theory-base accommodates any changes.

The learning sequence, initiated by a need for practice-based problem-solving, closes when the new theory is enmeshed in the new practice approach. Practice is then established, or affirmed, until the practitioner considers that this new approach has become unsatisfactory, when the whole process starts again.

The effective practitioner also needs to gain an understanding of wider organizational change and how this impacts on their practice and context. Blackler (1995) defines this as a crucial process for 'sense making' in an uncertain world. He suggests that this comprises:

- the need to understand fully the explicit structures of your particular organisation
- being able to analyse and predict the flow of organizational behaviour
- becoming adept at interpreting the significance of informal, implicit structures
- acknowledging the role played by knowledge production in change processes.

These four aspects will help the practitioner to understand their role in an organization and uncover the strategies and hidden agendas that impact upon their working context. There has been a tendency for nursing practice to deal with change by focusing on individual and behaviour change approaches. Primarily this has been via giving health advice to a 'captive' recipient – the patient. As Simnett (1995) notes, this is seldom effective (and often unethical) when considering the underlying ethos of equitable health-promoting practice.

Dealing with change needs to be grounded in a much wider political context. This is often difficult for those in a nursing context where the climate is often one of caution, conservatism and apparent 'apoliticism'. Many nurse practitioners view themselves as impervious to macropolitical issues, yet this approach itself may be construed as political positioning. The health-promoting nurse practitioner cannot ignore that the inequalities gap between richest and poorest in the UK is still growing and that poverty is the key predictor of poor quality of life, high morbidity and early death (Wilson-Barnett, 1993). Social, economic and political aspects impact on all facets of health promotion work. These aspects are then augmented by policy provision that reflects the prevailing dominant ideology.

Exercise

- How do social differentials impact on gastroenterology nursing?
- Why is the suggestion of becoming politically aware problematic in nursing?

The most productive use of a developed awareness occurs when wider issues of national and local policy can be assessed in relation to organizational and individual practice. Clearly, the impact of health restructuring that occurred in the early 1990s created dramatic changes for health and social care. Policies such as the NHS and Community Care

Act 1990 introduced the concept of 'purchasers' and 'providers' to health and social care provision. Its ethos was to make existing services more efficient and cost-effective, provide more choice for patients by freeing up the healthcare sector to private competition, become less bureaucratic and ultimately provide a better all-round system for patient care. As Jones and Sidell (1997) note, 'The reforms developed within a context of consumerism and market competition. There was a heavy emphasis on health care as an "industry" and on the patient as a health "consumer"' (p146). Since then, there has been a raft of other policies which have impacted on health-promoting practice, from the strictly targeted *Health of the Nation* (DoH, 1992) strategy to the New Labour approach of social responsibility underpinning both the *Our Healthier Nation* (DoH, 1999b) approach and the *Making a Difference* (DoH, 1999a) new NHS document.

Jones and Siddell (1997) identify four key stages that need to be critically evaluated in any policy-making processes:

- agenda setting: problem identification and issues recognition
- options development and appraisal: setting of alternatives, forecasting, cost:benefit analysis
- policy choice and implementation
- evaluation and review.

If the maxim of health promotion is to enable people to take more control over their own lives (WHO, 1986), then this may provide a useful evaluative template when applied to policy-making processes in working environments.

Exercise

Consider one of your local workplace policies.

- How many of the policy-making procedures involved all staff in active decision-making?
- When applying Ottawa Charter notions, how could policy processes have been more health promoting?

Evidence-based practice

This section considers the historical grounding of health-promoting practice in medical epidemiology. It also considers the sociocultural context of defining an 'acceptable' evidence base and discusses the need for practitioners to explore lay percepts of health. Problems of identifying and measuring success indicators in health promotion are examined alongside whether nursing should focus its health-promoting practice on salutogenesis or illness avoidance. This section concludes with assessing some of the difficulties involved in defining effective timescales for health-promoting practice in clinical settings.

The bulk of healthcare policy making is grounded in medical epidemiological justification, in which predictions regarding the population's health are used to prioritize where resources are placed. The emergent field of health-promoting practice has its historical roots in both epidemiology and nineteenth-century public health and sanitation concerns (fuelled by industrial benefactors who realized that a healthier workforce was also more productive!) (Ashton and Seymour, 1988). It is argued that the basis for medical epidemiology goes back even further – to the time of seventeenth-century philosopher René Descartes, who explored the relationship between mind and body. Descartes spawned a notion that became known as 'Cartesian dualism' (Flew, 1994), in which mind and body are two distinct systems. This idea was then utilized by medics from this period, providing medicine with a rather simplistic form of explanation – 'Cartesian analysis' – in which bodily wellness is no more than the effective functioning of its constituent parts. This produced the mechanistic approach, which still characterizes modern-day medicine: parts break down and are repaired or replaced in order to restore health.

Despite all the posturing regarding such 'evidence-based' practice, there is little concrete fact to support clear-cut relationships between cause and effect in healthcare. The tendency has been to link personal action to health outcome, yet for all the epidemiological research undertaken, no cohesive framework has emerged to demonstrate a clear association between specific risk factors and health-related behaviours (Clarke, 1993). This suggests that there is a clear need to refocus. Accepted epidemiological methods do not provide the fullest possible picture. People acquire information about their health from a variety of sources, which are then given validity. Traditional linear approaches limit the ways that causes, outcomes and patterns of illness are investigated (Lupton, 1997).

Many additional methodologies could be used alongside epidemiological analyses, especially given the complex nature of health per se. Information needs to be gathered by talking with people about the reality of their lives. Lay people possess considerable knowledge and understanding of their own health, which is often overlooked. Notions that lay people are often ignorant of medical matters relating to risk and lifestyle facets have not been upheld by research in this domain (Bury, 1994).

Despite this, much health-promoting practice is built on these spurious assumptions. Often, the delivery of highly selective risk information results in coercing individuals into reordering their own health priorities (Backett, 1992). This strategy fails to acknowledge that individuals already apply their own subjective reasoning to explaining personal health status (Lupton, 1995). This is determined by perceptions of 'lived' experience and sociocultural context, which combine to shape people's theories and expectations of both health and illness (Davison and Davey-Smith, 1995). Non-material cultural accounts emerge concerning luck, fate and randomness, which are commonly used to rationalize health status (Davison et al., 1992). Consequently, health information is often acted upon in a unique manner. Yet these lay percepts of health are not viewed as part of an acceptable evidence base.

The effective health-promoting practitioner needs to explore lay percepts of health and meld these with more 'traditional' views to gain a richer insight into health decision-making and action.

Exercise

- Who is a health 'expert'?
- Can patients be experts regarding their own health needs?
- Why are lay percepts of health often excluded from being part of an 'acceptable' evidence base?

Given the pressure that the NHS is under to be part of a 'best value' contract culture, the drive to create artificial constructs that purportedly measure effectiveness has escalated during the 1990s (Katz and Peberdy, 1997). The arrival of both QALY (quality-adjusted life years) and 'health gain' indicators has been at the expense of the more financially burdensome health need. This swing to outputs-based evidence of success rather than process means that health-promoting practice based on the 'feel-good' factor is no longer acceptable. Instead, an emphasis is now placed on funding forms of practice that will produce quantifiable and clearly measurable results. Defining success indicators in health promotion is often problematic due to its contested meaning. A salutogenic approach demands a range of complex process-based quality indicators as evidence of success, along with the application of medium- to long-term evaluation mechanisms (Katz and Peberdy, 1997). Due to very time-limited budgeting, health promotion initiatives are often expected to yield very specific short-term success indicators, making more holistic approaches completely unachievable. Even illness-avoidance approaches are difficult to measure in the short term, especially when linked to measuring habitual behaviour change or physical improvement that may take years to establish and is based on spurious cause and effect assumptions.

In a nursing context, providing health-promoting practice can be subject to considerable conflict and constraint. The desire to be 'health promoting' may be suppressed, especially when faced with lack of physical resources and strict time limits. Clearly, process-based forms of health promotion (built on client-centredness and individual empowerment notions) take time and considerable resourcing if they are to be established. The most realistic option for practitioners working in an acute nursing context is likely to involve making sure that patients receive good-quality health information based on their expressed needs. Practitioners need to be aware of the constraints of their particular working context and recognize the limits placed on their health-promoting role. Wilson-Barnett (1993) suggests that to be truly health promoting, nurses have to move away from focusing their attention on individuals and behaviour-change emphases. Doing what is achievable as effectively as possible is much better than having false and unrealistic expectations that are constantly frustrated.

Designing a health-promoting practice development plan

The following guidelines are provided to assist you in designing your own health-promoting practice development approach by helping with practical implementation of some of the theories explored in this chapter. This also relates to the exercises included to provide an opportunity for reflection in practice.

Generic suggestions for developing practice

Priority must be given to seeking patients' views of health. If your practice is to be patient-centred, then their self-defined needs should be given equal weight alongside any 'expert' needs and national priorities. Evidence-based practice should explore lay views in more depth: this may result in your becoming a research tool to facilitate your own clients needs.

Your practice should include a variety of approaches that enable you to promote health and respond to any subsequent changes. The latter may involve increasing knowledge and awareness, behavioural or environmental change, or policy formulation and implementation. The patient should be involved in decision-making processes at all stages of any health promotion initiative.

Inter-agency collaboration needs to be underpinned by a vision shared by all collaborators. Roles and contributions need to be clearly established and transparent to all. Intended and unintended outcomes should be measured at the same time as evaluating processes. This full and open dialogue will help to ensure that partnerships develop as effectively as possible.

Consideration needs to be given to reducing health inequalities through influencing both policy and practice, not through zealously adhering to individual behaviour-change approaches. Health professionals need to develop the fullest possible understanding of their particular organization's structures and functions. Only then will they be able to contribute towards policy and practice determination in an appropriate and realistic manner.

The ongoing evaluation and development of practice has to be a clear priority alongside other work-based tasks. Developmental mechanisms could include:

- reflections in practice
- undertaking overt and explicit process and outcome evaluations
- cultivating an expanding and dynamic evidence base.

The key factor in all these mechanisms centres around actively involving all parties (especially the patient) in these developmental processes and ongoing scrutiny.

Simnett (1995) provides a structured approach, useful for considering specific tasks required of particular individuals in their own working context. She suggests that effective implementation involves detailed planning and certain key elements.

Creating specific job-design development plans

There should be coherence with other jobs and tasks to ensure a significant contribution can be made to health promotion initiatives and services. Issues to consider include:

- whether health promotion is viewed as an 'add-on' service or integrated within everyday practice

- whether it is adequately resourced and given appropriate validity alongside therapeutic, curative and acute provision.

Consideration should be given to utilizing a range of methods and skills, dependent on the overall context of the initiative. Issues to consider include:

- establishing how many different approaches are used in the context of your health-promoting practice
- whether you rely primarily on leaflets and posters, when changing the overall environment may be more appropriate and effective.

Employees should have considerable control and responsibility over how tasks are carried out and interpreted. Issues to consider include:

- whether the practitioner has any real autonomy of practice
- taking time to evaluate your own contribution in any health promotion initiatives, alongside any overall success.

Continuous assessment of job development processes needs to be part of any job-design programme. Issues to consider include:

- whether there are inbuilt opportunities for ongoing development of both knowledge and practice change
- recognizing that change processes are dynamic, not static, and that your own health-promoting role is regularly reviewed to take this into account.

This chapter has attempted to inform an understanding of health-promoting practice that corresponds to the overall ethos of patient-centredness underpinning this book. As suggested, health-promoting practice for the gastroenterology practitioner must be underpinned by realism and by prioritizing specific elements of practice as dictated by achievable needs. This chapter has explored:

1 the phenomenon of patient-centred practice and differing interpretations
2 constraints and opportunities for collaborative working
3 escalating change processes and the capacity to address these
4 the possible uses and abuses of evidence-based practice

5 possible templates for constructing and implementing a practice
   development plan.

This is summarized by Macleod Clark (1993), who defines the particular
characteristics desirable for 'health nursing' as: collaborative,
individualized, negotiated, supportive and (perhaps most crucially)
facilitative of healthcare.

References

Abbott SA (1998) Patient education: pre- and post-procedure upper endoscopy.
    Gastroenterology Nursing 22(1), 14–17.
Albrecht G, Freeman S, Higginbotham N (1998) Complexity and human health: the case for a
    trans-disciplinary paradigm. Culture, Medicine and Psychiatry 22(1), 55–92.
Antonovsky A (1993) The sense of coherence as a determinant of health. In: Beattie A, Gott M,
    Jones L, Sidell M (eds) Health and Wellbeing: a reader. Basingstoke: Macmillan.
Ashton J, Seymour H (1988) The New Public Health. Milton Keynes: Open University Press.
Backett K (1992) Taboos and excesses: lay health moralities in middle class families. Sociology
    of Health and Illness 14, 255–274.
Ball E (1998) Exercise guidelines for patients with inflammatory bowel disease.
    Gastroenterology Nursing 21(3), 108–111.
Beattie A (1991) Knowledge and control in health promotion: a test case for social policy and
    social theory. In: Gabe J, Calnan M, Bury M (eds) The Sociology of the Health Service.
    London: Routledge.
Blackler F (1995) Knowledge, knowledge work and organisations: an overview and
    interpretation. Organization Studies 16(6), 1021–1046.
Bury M (1994) Health promotion and lay epidemiology: a sociological view. Health Care
    Analysis 2(3), 23–30.
Campbell T (1998) Patient-focused care: primary responsibilities of research nurses. British
    Journal of Nursing 7(22), 1405–1409.
Caplan R, Holland R (1990) Rethinking health education theory. Health Education Journal
    49(1), 10–12.
Clarke JB (1993) Ethical issues in health education. British Journal of Nursing 2(10), 533–537.
Davison C, Davey-Smith G (1995) The baby and the bath water: examining socio-cultural and
    free-market critiques of health promotion. In: Bunton R, Nettleton S, Burrows R (eds) The
    Sociology of Health Promotion: critical analyses of consumption, lifestyle and risk. London:
    Routledge.
Davison C, Frankel LS, Davey-Smith G (1992) The limits of lifestyle: reassessing 'fatalism' in
    the popular culture of illness prevention. Social Science and Medicine 34(6), 675–685.
Department of Health (1989) Working for Patients. London: HMSO.
Department of Health (1992) The Health of the Nation. London: HMSO.
Department of Health (1997) The New NHS: modern, dependable. London: DoH.
Department of Health (1998a) The Acheson Report. London: DoH.
Department of Health (1998b) Smoking Kills. London: DoH.
Department of Health (1999a) Making a Difference: strengthening the nursing, midwifery and
    health visiting contribution to health and health care. London: DoH.
Department of Health (1999b) Saving Lives: our healthier nation. London: DoH.

Ewles L, Simnett E (1999) Promoting Health: a practical guide, 4th edn. Edinburgh: Baillière Tindall.

Flew A (1994) A Dictionary of Philosophy, 2nd edn. London: Pan Books.

Forster D (1995) Groups and teams. In: Pike S, Forster D (eds) Health Promotion for All. Edinburgh: Churchill Livingstone.

Gottlieb LN, Gottlieb B (1998) Evolutionary principles can guide nursing's future development. Journal of Advanced Nursing 28(5), 1099–1105.

Griffiths R (1983) NHS Management Inquiry. London: Department of Health and Social Security.

Ham C (1999) Health Policy in Britain, 4th edn. Basingstoke: Macmillan.

Handy C (1991) Gods of Management, 3rd edn. London: Business Books.

HMSO (1990) National Health Service and Community Care Act. London: HMSO.

Joint Committee of Professional Nursing, Midwifery and Health Visiting Associations (England) (1997) A Celebration of Nursing, Midwifery and Health Visiting: essential ingredients of health care. London: Joint Committee of Professional Nursing, Midwifery and Health Visiting Associations (England).

Jones L (1997) What is health? In: Katz J, Peberdy A (eds) Promoting Health: knowledge and practice. Basingstoke: Macmillan.

Jones L, Naidoo J (1997) Theories and models in health promotion. In: Katz J, Peberdy A (eds) Promoting Health: knowledge and practice. Basingstoke: Macmillan.

Jones L, Sidell M (eds) (1997) The Challenge of Promoting Health: exploration and action. Buckingham: Open University.

Katz J, Peberdy A (eds) (1997) Promoting Health: knowledge and practice. Basingstoke: Macmillan.

Latter S (1998) Health promotion in the acute setting. In: Kendall S (ed) Health and Empowerment Research and Practice. London: Arnold.

Leathard A (1997) Collaboration: united we stand, divided we fall? In: Jones L, Sidell M (eds) The Challenge of Promoting Health: exploration and action. Buckingham: Open University.

Lupton D (1995) The Imperative of Health: public health and the regulated body. London: Sage.

Lupton D (1997) Epidemiology as a socio-cultural practice. Critical Public Health 7(1 & 2), 28–37.

Macleod Clark J (1993) From sick nursing to health nursing evolution or revolution? In: Wilson-Barnett J, Macleod Clark J (eds) Research in Health Promotion and Nursing. Basingstoke: Macmillan.

Maynard A (1995) Is killing people wrong? Health Service Journal 26 January, 21.

Meyer J (1993) Lay participation in care: threat to the status quo? In: Wilson-Barnett J, Macleod Clark J (eds) Research in Health Promotion and Nursing. Basingstoke: Macmillan.

McBride A (1995) Health Promotion in Hospital: a practical handbook for nurses. London: Scutari Press.

Naidoo J, Wills J (1998) Practising Health Promotion: dilemmas and challenges. London: Baillière Tindall.

Ovretveit J (1993) Coordinating Community Care: multi-disciplinary teams and care management. Buckingham: Open University Press.

Pike S (1995) What is health promotion? In: Pike S, Forster D (eds) Health Promotion for All. Edinburgh: Churchill Livingstone.

Robinson S, Hill Y (1998) The health promoting nurse. Journal of Clinical Nursing 7, 232–238.

Ross H (1998) Constipation: cause and control in an acute hospital setting. British Journal of Nursing 7(15), 907–913.

Saddler DA (1999) Education for the gastroenterology cancer patient. Gastroenterology Nursing 22(3), 122–125.

Schon DA (1983) The Reflective Practitioner: how professionals think in action. New York: Basic Books.

Sidell M (1997) Partnerships and collaboration; the promise of participation. In: Jones L, Sidell M (eds) The Challenge of Promoting Health: exploration and action. Buckingham: Open University.

Simnett I (1995) Managing Health Promotion: developing healthy organisations and communities. Chichester: Wiley.

Skinner J (1995) Towards an integrated model of health promotion in nursing practice. In: Pike S, Forster D (eds) Health Promotion for All. Edinburgh: Churchill Livingstone.

Smolen DM, Topp R (1997) Coping methods of patients with inflammatory bowel disease and prediction of perceived health, functional status, and well-being. Gastroenterology Nursing 21(3), 112–118.

Tones K, Tilford S, Robinson Y (1990) Health Education: effectiveness and efficiency. London: Chapman and Hall.

United Kingdom Council for Nursing, Midwifery and Health Visiting (1992) Code of Professional Conduct for Nurses, Midwives and Health Visitors, 2nd edn. London: UKCC.

Wilson-Barnett J (1993) Health promotion and nursing practice. In: Dines A, Cribb A (eds) Health Promotion: concepts and practice. Oxford: Blackwell Science.

Wilson-Barnett J, Latter S (1993) Factors influencing nurses' health education and health promotion practice in acute ward areas. In: Wilson-Barnett J, Macleod Clark J (eds) Research in Health Promotion and Nursing. Basingstoke: Macmillan Press.

Woodward VM (1998) Caring, patient autonomy and the stigma of paternalism. Journal of Advanced Nursing 28(5), 1046–1052.

World Health Organization (1985) Health For All in Europe by the Year 2000 – regional targets. Copenhagen: WHO.

World Health Organization (1986) Ottawa Charter for Health Promotion. Copenhagen: WHO.

CHAPTER 9
Ethics

JAMES M MERCER

Introduction

This chapter demystifies ethics by considering the nature and relevance of ethics to professional clinical practice. It is intended to persuade readers of the importance of ethics with reference to accountability and autonomy linked to the challenge posed by patients having 'interests'. The overall intention of this chapter is to focus readers' attention on the place and importance of ethics in clinical practice as an effective and essential means of developing and expanding proactive clinical responsibility. The chapter ends with an exercise designed to support the reader in applying theory to practice.

The ethical dimension

Practice without theory is futile.
Theory without practice is mere intellectual play.
I Kant (1724–1804), cited in Dworkin (1988)

The intention of this chapter is to illuminate readers' appreciation concerning the value of ethics in healthcare. This value is reflected in the skilled utilization and development of critical analysis, which lies at the heart of ethical activity. Thinking hard about issues in a disciplined and informed way is often difficult and demanding. The uncertainty it arouses can be uncomfortable, but ensures one against the dangers of moral complacency. Critical analysis transcends professional boundaries and is a significant feature in all forms of professional activity. The view of ethics as a 'core' element in this book highlights the fact that all healthcare professionals must develop the ethical dimensions of their role if they intend to be taken seriously in multidisciplinary clinical environments.

Many nurses in clinical practice still fail to take ethics seriously in their everyday work, regarding the matter as merely theoretical debate for academic colleagues. Ethics in healthcare is often criticized by assuming it means having to acquire obscure moral theories linked with the ability to speak in a largely incomprehensible fashion (Hunt, 1994). Those who hold this view also tend to believe that such 'exclusive' activity devalues personally held morality, obliging the ordinary professional to approach ethical activity 'empty handed'. Nothing could be further from the truth, because it is the very ordinariness of personally held moral views that feeds ethical debate, infusing it with a dynamic in contrast to an inert character. Ethics has to be regarded as a lived experience not as some fossilized curiosity, which has long ceased to have any relevance to the human condition. The very act of thinking seriously about what concerns you as an individual confirms the validity of ethical reflection.

The relevance of ethics is often characterized by a form of neutrality, which means that no single individual or organization can lay claim to a monopoly of superior ethical belief and behaviour. Neutrality ends when interpretation of ethical views and opinions begins, and what is important concerns the critical examination of those views and opinions. It may appear that the medical profession lays claim to a monopoly in the NHS, but this is only because other healthcare professionals such as nurses have allowed this illusion to masquerade as reality. I believe this state of affairs has helped to reinforce in the nursing consciousness the assumption that medical 'moral' opinion must always be viewed as synonymous with 'professional' medical opinion. This attitude has tended to maintain nursing moral opinion in a defensive position. Nurses who hold this view understandably exhibit a spectrum of defensive responses towards ethics, believing that a fragmented relationship exists between ethics and practical bedside nursing. The rest of this chapter is dedicated to the unpackaging and demystifying of these implications and their meaning.

The terms 'ethics' and 'moral philosophy' will be used interchangeably throughout this chapter.

I intend to offer an exploration of the nature and meaning of ethics and its relevance to healthcare professionals in general and registered nurses in particular. I have chosen to focus on a narrow range, which I hope will be sufficient to convince readers of this relevance. Through this exploration I want to identify the moral implications for nurses who are setting out to develop their professional roles into areas of potential ambiguity and conflict. It is not intended, nor would it be feasible in a work of this nature, to explore such issues in a rigorously exhaustive way. The focus will be on implications for practice, which will hopefully encourage readers towards the deeper end of ethical thinking and debate. In using this approach I wish to encourage readers to consider an integrated view of the moral issues as they apply to the context of good nursing and thereby come to a self-realization that ethical theory and clinical practice are indeed inextricably interwoven.

The meaning of ethics

Every day, nurses in practice exercise judgement and emotion (feelings) in specific contexts, attempting to create morally good options. This democratic understanding of ethical behaviour is validated by Gillon (1989), who offers what I think to be a particularly useful definition of moral philosophy (ethics):

> An analytic activity in which concepts, assumptions, beliefs, attitudes, emotions, reasons and arguments underlying medicomoral decision-making are examined critically (p5).

This definition is clearly rooted in the human condition, with all its complexities and contradictions. For example, consider for a moment your own assumptions, beliefs, attitudes and emotions concerning the allocation of limited healthcare resources. Through a process of critical reflection, applying Gillon's definition of ethics one may gain a clearer insight into *why* a particular view is held. This process can be unsettling, as it may point towards the need to change or moderate long-cherished personal views. Submitting oneself to such a process enables a more meaningful dialogue to take place when one extends Gillon's definition to challenge other professionals' concepts, assumptions and beliefs.

It is not uncommon for unrehearsed and uninformed views concerning moral questions to create feelings of personal threat. There is then a tendency to demonize other people for the views they hold, which shuts off any meaningful access to understanding why such viewpoints are held. It must be noted that in understanding another's moral point of view one is not obliged to automatically accept such a view in place of one's own. By understanding others' viewpoints one learns to move away from simplistic assumptions of what is morally right or wrong. The focus moves towards a critical analysis of moral choices and in this context helps to discover a deeper appreciation of rightness/wrongness in moral acts.

In the 5th century BC, the Athenian philosopher Socrates showed that, by asking persistent and often abrasive questions, the easy confidence with which individuals often hold on to personal opinions concerning moral matters is not always matched by their understanding of them (Jackson, 1992). In medico-moral debate this ability to ask questions is refined and raised to a higher level of intellectual activity in which all healthcare professionals have an obligation to take a full part. The practical application of this ability liberates the individual healthcare professional from the often fruitless search for 'the right answer' concerning the dilemmas and challenges posed by everyday professional life. The credibility of moral philosophy in clinical practice does not arise from the measured use of some abstract moral rhetoric. It arises from the associated weight of reason that is employed to inform ethical behaviour. This crucial assertion enables the practitioner to transcend professional boundaries, enabling the application of critical analysis to be focused on all forms of argument and debate. In utilizing this approach, ethics does not provide universal answers but does seek to offer a 'pathway' for reasoned thought (Kendrick, 1993).

It is stated in published literature with perennial regularity that nursing is a practice-based profession. Nowadays, nurses working in academia would no doubt enthusiastically join in the general chorus of this declaration, but equally declare that ethics applied to healthcare forms an integral part of this practice. Ethics, or more properly moral philosophy, and professional healthcare are inextricably connected if one is committed to good nursing practice (Elliott-Pennels, 1999).

Historically, nurses' education emphasized a hierarchical and task-oriented approach, training and moulding individuals to behave reactively in clinical practice. A significant consequence of this approach for nurses' professional activity was reflected by their expectation of finding 'the answer' to problems or the 'correct way' of carrying out procedures with numerical precision. This passive educational approach often denied to nurses the ability to develop enquiring minds, pose challenging questions and the means to think independently. This chapter is offered as a useful means of enhancing professional self-confidence and of encouragement to translate such thinking into proactive clinical practice.

It is of paramount importance that nurses come to realize that the most effective means of moderating what they may see as inappropriate medico-moral decision-making is by proactively engaging in rational and focused dialogue, which constructively challenges the medico-moral decision-making process. Such dialogue demands attention to be maintained on the interests of the patient, and in this essential activity, far from being ethically marginalized, nurses have a unique role to play (Moores, 1999). For this reason, I am most concerned that, in terms of their analytical skills, readers acquire a mature appreciation of moral philosophy (ethics).

The skills of moral analysis are an indispensable part of the repertoire of healthcare professionals practising in diverse, complex and multidisciplinary environments. Ethical activity ought to be viewed as an ordinary part of practical, everyday healthcare delivery. It is only by engaging this route that the true worth of ethics can be cherished, not only by nurses, but by all healthcare professionals who place the interests of patients first. This common ground ought to be viewed as a source of reassurance by nurses. Such reassurance offers compelling evidence that, far from being an exclusive activity, ethics in healthcare demands the inclusion of all professionals, not just a chosen few.

The question of 'interests'

When challenged to explain what it means to act in a patient's best interests, most healthcare professionals are unable to offer an adequate explanation. First, we need to consider what it means to have interests. For example, one could say that a stone does not have interests since nothing we can do could harm it (Singer, 1986). In this example, Singer seems to be suggesting that some level of consciousness is required in order to have interests. In person-centred activity like healthcare, this criterion fails to include those times when otherwise conscious beings are asleep or unconscious (Ellis, 1996). The implications of failure to include the interests of such beings are clear to any right-thinking healthcare professional. For example, the 'safety' of an unconscious patient for any right-thinking nurse surely forms an integral part of nursing care. The patient may be in an unconscious state, but this does not cancel out their moral interests.

The focus of 'interest' in the healthcare context is best understood by a consideration of individuals' well-being. As the philosopher Bentham once said: 'The question is not can they reason but can they suffer?' Dworkin (1993) suggests that it is only pleasurable or painful experiences that can or cannot be in our best interests. Part of his theory focuses on 'critical interests' and includes those features that make life worthwhile, such as love, beauty and friendship. Dworkin states:

> We need an intellectual explanation of critical interests, so that we may better understand these ideas from the inside, understand introspectively how they connect with other large beliefs we have about life and death and why human life has intrinsic worth.

Although critical interests are difficult to define precisely, it is reasonable to suggest that they include many of the features such as dignity and respect, which form what may be termed a 'good life'. They relate to the way in which individuals choose to lead their lives and many would argue they retain their importance even if a person is unaware or in an unconscious state (Feinberg, 1974). The idea that professionals ought to protect and promote the critical interests of individuals even though the individual concerned may be unaware is of vital importance because it involves trust, which is a key moral issue inextricably bound up with human relationships. It is well to recall that in terms of any human relationship, once trust is betrayed the consequences can be very damaging, depending on the level of harm generated by the betrayal.

Consider the following example where a woman goes into a police station to report a serious sexual assault. The police officer concerned with her case takes her into a room where he photographs her nude on the premiss that such photographs will be needed as evidence if the case goes to court. However, instead of using the photographs for evidence, he passes them around his colleagues. The woman is unaware of this occurrence, and it could be argued that since she is unaware of the illicit act of the police officer she has not suffered 'harm'. However, it is clear that the officer has not acted in the 'best critical interests' of the woman (Rachels, 1991). The standard required of professionals to protect the critical interests of individuals is an exacting one and does not cease simply because the individual may not be aware of our actions.

Moral philosophy is a complicated matter but complexity per se cannot be used as a reason for not engaging in moral thought. Professional practice in healthcare is also well recognized as a complicated matter. The most cursory inspection of UKCC published literature will reveal this fact (e.g. Guidelines for Professional Practice). Clinical nursing practice can be greatly enhanced if one accepts the proposition that both moral philosophy and professional practice are concerned with judgement and decision-making.

This involves having the right feeling at the right time and recognizing that each occasion is different (Warnock, 1998). This approach acknowledges the value of ethics to a person-centred activity like nursing. It also raises awareness of shared interests where complex and demanding challenges are accepted as the norm.

Such challenges require attention to be directed towards a meaningful consideration of morally appropriate choices based on a well-founded rationale. When viewed in this light, the moral self-examination based on

Gillon's definition can be extended to the examination of other healthcare professionals' beliefs, attitudes and emotions. Persistent questioning, using the Socratic model, enables the cultivation of moral dialogue among diverse healthcare professionals, creating a climate of reasonable and rational moral co-operation. This approach ultimately protects and serves the best interests of the 'patient' by making it possible to provide an acceptable level of 'seamless service' in the delivery of professional healthcare (Moores, 1999).

In exercising critical analysis within a moral perspective, it becomes self-evident that far from approaching 'empty handed', each healthcare professional brings to the moral debate a sophisticated personal collection of assumptions, beliefs, attitudes and emotions. This collection is often born out of the costly personal experiences of daily living and the necessity of having to face the ethical demands associated with such experience. In this light, moral activity can be appreciated as a continuous process, a creative struggle in which moral options and their associated cost are confronted and considered. Such cost can range from feeling a certain unease about a particular decision, to what is often referred to as whistle blowing. The Graham Pink affair is a particularly clear example of whistle blowing, where an individual nurse felt his duty to serve the public interest ultimately outweighed the duty owed to his employer. By reflecting on this continuous process, nurses are enabled to place a perspective on the responsibility for the personal choices ultimately made and retain a measure of control over events.

Accountability/autonomy

The role of the nurse has significantly changed over recent years, reflecting the rapidly changing demands associated with the NHS (Smith, 1995). Such demands have directly influenced the increasing development of a professional identity, and one of the societal demands associated with this status concerns the production of a 'code' (Willard, 1996).

The Code of Professional Conduct (UKCC, 1992) alerts healthcare professionals to their responsibilities by laying down certain rules and principles, which reflect the standard of professional and moral behaviour expected of every registered practitioner. The generic nature of codes poses a major challenge for practitioners covered by such a document. For example, the Code of Professional Conduct states: 'act always in such a manner as to promote and safeguard the interests and well-being of patients and clients' (Clause 1). The challenge of a universal statement like this lies in its application to the diverse and specific clinical contexts within which the registered practitioner exercises his or her role. Rules and principles such as those contained in codes are useful as well-grounded guidance. But the subjective judgement of the individual practitioner in specific contexts has to be supported as 'ultimate' (Seedhouse, 1998). Because of the key principle that every practitioner be personally accountable for his or her individual actions, the interpretation and application of principles/rules must ultimately be a subjective act.

We hear a good deal today about the autonomous practitioner, but in reality very few nurses, if any, can claim to occupy such a role. Technological advances have also had considerable influence on the definition and meaning of professional nursing roles. The nature of such advances has required nurses to assume ever-greater levels of responsibility. Unfortunately, the official authority or recognition, which such levels of responsibility normally command, has often been denied to these nurses (Ellis and Hartley, 1988). This state of affairs poses a central question, which any nurse considering assuming greater levels of responsibility must carefully reflect on before choosing a course of action:

> Whether nurses be considered to have the professional judgement and training to decide what activities they are qualified to undertake, or whether this decision should be taken by others?
>
> (Ward, 1991, p35).

Ward identifies the 'others' referred to in this quotation as the 'medical profession'. The implication reflects a signal for nurses to actively engage medical colleagues and clinical management in the creation of written protocols/contracts. The aim must be to minimize the inherent risks associated with ambiguity of professional responsibilities.

Autonomy has its origins in reference to the self-rule or self-governance of the Greek city states. This original meaning was then applied to individuals, and given moral status by Kant (cited in Dworkin, 1988). In common usage, it implies 'being one's own person or being able to act according to one's beliefs or desires without interference'. It thus requires the capacity to think rationally and to make a reasoned decision consistent with one's values, and the ability to think and act freely, without undue influence from others (Clarke, 1999).

Vitally important questions arise when nurses begin to extend and expand their professional boundaries, in particular, questions surrounding the relationship between accountability and autonomy when associated with changing roles. The UKCC (1992) clearly states that nurses must be responsible and accountable for their actions and work from an autonomous base. However, the term 'autonomous base' is not defined in the document; neither is there any indication at what level the principle ought to operate. In order to be autonomous, the practitioner must have the ability to determine professional boundaries and limitations. For others to be allowed to determine these matters undermines the whole raison d'être of what it means to be an autonomous practitioner, if we consider the contribution of Clarke (1999). Autonomy will always require moderation because of the fact that nurses have a commitment to each member of the team with whom they work. Therefore, the possession and development of autonomy will always require careful thought and rational dialogue with colleagues in order to establish credibility and professional boundaries of accountability.

This is especially true when undertaking and developing new roles in the delivery of healthcare. The implications in terms of accountability can be profound. It requires a certain kind of courage to assume accountability for a role whose nature has largely been determined by *other* healthcare professionals. The well-understood term 'fall guy' comes to mind where professional responsibility is offered without an equal measure of power and control over the necessary resources. In such circumstances, nurses can find themselves being held to account for decisions taken by others.

Seedhouse (1998) offers a view of autonomy very much in tune with contemporary professional nursing practice. He asserts autonomy as essentially a quality, by stating, 'to be autonomous is to be able to do' (p182). This approach potentially offers the professional nurse a feasible autonomous base from which to develop specialist clinical roles. An essential prerequisite concerns a careful exploration of the deceptively simple question: able to do what? Irrespective of the answer, one element is clear – nurses must make certain they have a major say in determining the boundaries and limitations of any changes to their professional practice. This is particularly important when one considers such authors as Mitchinson (1996), who carefully considered the independence and autonomy of the modern nurse and stated:

> It is deemed doubtful, however, if any of the nurses currently working in hospital, community or general practice are autonomous and independent (p7).

Mitchinson based this conclusion on the nature of existing power structures within the NHS and the status of other health professionals and managers. I suggest that the development of healthcare professionals possessing high levels of autonomy would prove personally threatening to existing structures of power and control. It is clear from any review of the literature that, in the present political and economic climate, what cannot be controlled is often viewed as a threat. The way forward for the appropriately motivated nurse in such a climate involves defining and setting her own parameters within a context of adequate education, training and trust. This represents the only meaningful route, which will bring about a true sense of autonomy for the nursing profession (Mitchinson, 1996).

The moral implications for nurses in the present healthcare climate are rooted in the necessity to take control of the autonomous development and expansion of their professional role. In this climate, conflict and ambiguity are ever present and nurses must therefore initially safeguard and promote their own interests before they will be in a position to do the same for patients. For many years it has been asserted that nursing should be seeking professionalism through improved care for patients and clients, and not higher status for 'ourselves' (Downe, 1990). Higher professional status attracts authority and it is only through the recognition of this authority by both society and other healthcare professionals that improved patient care can be achieved. The nature of this 'authority' is traditionally grounded in carefully thought-out rationale and informed ethical argument. If a lack of professional authority is allowed to develop, serious fault lines can undermine the whole venture. For example, senior clinical nurses often find they are holding responsibility for standards without the means to achieve and raise them. This familiar scenario leads to uncomfortable levels of compromise concerning personal and professional moral principles. This is why viewing ethical activity and the skills associated with critical analysis are so important. Unless nurses are able to engage colleagues in rational and informed argument, their ability to influence and moderate medico-moral decision-making will be seriously hampered.

The professional development and expansion of roles also entails the challenge to create a balance between the skills associated with technological advances and traditional nursing practice. The cost of getting this balance wrong means the erosion of nursing identity in a multidisciplinary working environment where the role of the nurse is eventually replaced by roles such as 'physician's assistant' (Norris, 1995).

Conclusion

I hope this chapter encourages readers to embark on their professional development with a revitalized understanding in terms of the ethical dimensions, and a curiosity to read and think more deeply of future roles. I am sure Rudyard Kipling would excuse my parody of the last lines of his popular poem 'If':

> If you can keep your head when all about you is chaos and confusion you must be a nurse!

Exercise 1

Imagine at some time in the future you are offered a clinical post as a specialist nurse. Prior to taking up the appointment you ask to discuss the details of the terms and conditions of your potential new employment with the human resource manager and the senior medical clinician with whom you will be working on a daily basis.

Take into account the key elements that have been included in this chapter, namely: critical thinking, the question of interests (your own and patients), accountability, influence over resources and professional autonomy.

Consider how you might put an agenda together utilizing these elements so that in terms of the ethical, legal and professional issues, you ensure that your contribution to the discussion is taken seriously and is reflected in the final contract.

Exercise 2

List the ethical considerations that apply in gastroenterological nursing practice to:

- you as a professional
- the patient.

Consider the ethical framework you will practise within, utilizing the elements discussed in this chapter relating to accountability, autonomy, ethical, legal and professional issues.

References

Clarke DM (1999) Autonomy, rationality and the wish to die. Journal of Medical Ethics 25, 475–662.

Downe SA (1990) A noble vocation. Nursing Times 86(24), 40

Dworkin R (1988) The Theory and Practice of Autonomy. Cambridge: Cambridge University Press.

Dworkin R (1993) Life's Dominion: an argument about abortion and euthanasia. London: Harper-Collins.

Elliott-Pennels C (1999) The essence of nursing. Nursing Standard 1 (23), 42–46.

Ellis P (1996) Exploring the concept of acting 'in the patient's best interests'. British Journal of Nursing 5(17), 1072–1074.

Ellis J, Hartley C (1988) Nursing in Today's World. Challenges, issues and trends, 3rd edn. Philadelphia, Pa: Lippincott.

Feinberg J (1974) The rights of animals and unborn generations. In: Blackstone W (ed) Philosophy and Environmental Crisis. University of Georgia Press.

Gillon R (1989) Philosophical Medical Ethics. Chichester: Wiley and Sons.

Hunt G (1994) What is nursing ethics? Nurse Education Today 12 October, 323–328.

Jackson J (1992) Coming to ethical terms 'Ethics'. Business Ethics: European Review 1(1), 1–3.

Kendrick K (1993) Understanding ethics in nursing practice. British Journal of Nursing 12(18), 920–925.

Mitchinson S (1996) Are nurses independent and autonomous practitioners? Nursing Standard 10(34), 34–39.

Moores Y (1999) Nurses are 'powerhouse' for better quality NHS. Department of Health 1999/0632.

Norris E (1995) Achieving professional autonomy for nursing. Professional Nurse 11(1), 59–61.

Rachels J (1991) In: White J (ed.) Contemporary Moral Problems. New York: West Publishing.

Seedhouse D (1998) Ethics: the heart of healthcare. Chichester: Wiley and Sons.

Singer P (1986) Applied Ethics. Cambridge: Cambridge University Press.

Smith C (1995) Evaluating nursing care: reflection in practice. Professional Nurse 10(11), 723–734.

UKCC (1992) Code of Professional Conduct, 2nd edn. London: UKCC.

Ward R (1991) The extended role of the nurse: a review. Nursing Standard 6(11), 33–36.

Warnock M (1998) An Intelligent Person's Guide to Ethics. London: Duckworth.

Willard C (1996) The nurse's role as patient advocate: obligation or imposition? Journal of Advanced Nursing 24(1), 60–66.

CHAPTER 10

Professional judgement and clinical decision-making

DIANE PALMER

Introduction

The process of professional judgement cannot be prescribed. The application of judgement to aid decision-making is a process that must be learnt, as it is based on challenge and uncertainty, and is unique to the situation of the time (Girot, 2000). We learn from an early age to apply judgements and make decisions, supported by rules and guidance. I am sure that many of us as children learnt that it is dangerous to cross the road, but often necessary and at times unavoidable. The associated risks, however, can be significantly reduced if some basic rules are followed, such as looking right and left and right again, and if there is no approaching traffic in the near vicinity it is assumed safe to start to cross the road. Judgement, however, must be applied to the situation if, while crossing the road, a vehicle is seen or heard and appears to be approaching quickly. Do you turn back or keep going to the other side? Similar principles can be applied to most situations; basic rules and guidelines will support you in decision-making once you are familiar with the presenting circumstances, although should the situation change or events not go according to plan, then a degree of judgement must be applied. However, in situations such as healthcare, the judgement and decision should be calculated against any potential risks and must be justifiable.

The aim of this chapter is to provide guidance for nurses that can be incorporated into decision-making in the clinical environment. A nurse cannot rely on the defence of simply taking action because a doctor or senior member of staff has ordered it. She must be able to justify every action taken and decision made, while having the ability to apply logic and clinical reasoning to any judgements made.

Critical thinking, defined as the ability to problem solve by analysis of information, logical thinking and formulation of conclusions (Bandman and Bandman, 1988; Watson and Glaser, 1991), is essential for the autonomous practitioner promoting safety, competency, skill and effectiveness (Jones and Brown, 1991). 'In my professional experience' is an expression often used by healthcare staff who are advising patients faced with treatment options. The advice offered, however, is not simply based on what has been seen in practice over a series of years (although this information is significantly utilized in the decision-making equation). Also required is a sound collation of knowledge stored in a systematic form and called upon to support the decision-making and guide the judgements.

The processes involved in making judgements and decisions do utilize similar information, but do not necessarily produce the same outcome. A judgement is passive, it is merely the provision of knowledge. However, a decision usually initiates or terminates action.

Decision analysis

When attempting to solve a clinical diagnostic problem, the first stage is identification of the problem and then, second, the cause needs to be determined. Certain signs, such as pyrexia or obesity, may be easy to recognize and measure, while others, such as a rash or symptoms of occasional pain or abdominal bloating, may be harder to identify and categorize. Not all of the information required to make a diagnosis will be available and the practitioner must determine which issues to explore and which to ignore. Therefore, the next stage in the decision-making process is to draft a plan of data to be collected and considered, from which inferences can be drawn. This is necessary, as not every patient will present in the same manner complaining of the same severity or range of symptoms and signs, so a picture has to be built. Additionally, other issues, such as social and moral factors, should be considered and, depending on their relevance, taken into account.

In the search for a diagnosis, consideration of any proposed investigations should include benefits, risks, costs, side effects and inconvenience, with a balance being sought between patient preferences and consequences and benefits of treatment. When discussing options, always remember that the decision to do nothing is a decision in itself, as it supports the current situation (Bandman and Bandman, 1988) and as such has to be justified, and of course it will be an appropriate choice in many instances. It should also be remembered that people have different concepts of success. The option of 'the best operation that money can buy' may be a favoured option for some people but a feared and unrealistic option for others. There is little point in requesting expensive, sophisticated investigations if all the outcomes require, for example, surgical intervention or pharmaceutical therapy, which the patient is not fit enough to tolerate.

Decision analysis does assume that people have fairly well-defined preferences. However, in practice, it has been found that when faced with complex and sensitive options, the original preferences can be difficult to maintain (Eraker and Politser, 1982). Over time and with pressure, original values get distorted, therefore it is important to be aware that a person may change his or her mind or choose alternative preferences, which may even have been previously disregarded. This, of course, can be a major problem when trying to consider options in line with the values of an individual.

Another problem in decision analysis is the issue of how far into the future to consider when discussing treatment options (Eraker and Sox, 1981), particularly when you are aware that over time people change their minds. Therefore, any decisions made or judgements applied should be regularly reassessed or reconsidered, either in light of new and/or additional information or circumstances, or simply the passage of time.

Clinical reasoning and inference

Clinical reasoning is the thinking and decision-making process applied in clinical practice. Problem solving in clinical practice involves decision-making in a critical, analytical and autonomous manner. Core elements required are the use of knowledge, the act of thinking and meta-cognition: the awareness of knowledge and consideration in thought processes. Increased knowledge and technological assistance has enhanced the complexity of the decision-maker's task in the clinical environment (Dowie and Elstein, 1988), with the whole approach requiring effective information-processing skills.

Clinical reasoning is the process that supports decision-making, as it formulates meanings for observed situations. Situational cues are used to make intuitive inferences, by selectively processing information to formulate hypotheses which can be tested. Clinical reasoning skills can be learnt by supervised practice, with progressive increase in responsibility, and supported by clinical teaching and supervision. This process can be very effective as it allows analysis and discussion, although it is time-consuming.

Inferential reasoning has to be applied to data received according to the circumstances, which can be cognitively demanding. Indeed, not all clinicians have the appropriate skills to process new information (Gambrill, 1990) and apply inferential reasoning, therefore tools and models such as algorithms and flow charts have to be utilized, which indicate pathways of care to be followed. Experienced clinicians, however, can formulate a working hypothesis or diagnosis within 15 seconds of a conversation with a patient (Elstein et al., 1978). Case conferences, ward rounds, reading and literature review all help to develop skills in clinical and diagnostic reasoning, although time and experience contribute extensively.

Assessment in relation to patients' needs

The patient must have appropriate involvement for reliable, effective decision-making to take place. One of the primary aims should be to establish the patient's knowledge and feeling about the illness and prognosis. The practitioner must be aware of the patient's perception of the risks and/or benefits of any tests or treatment being offered, to enable their attitudes and beliefs to be taken into account in the judgement in order that the natural sense of the situation can be incorporated.

When considering diagnostic intervention, this should always be in the best interests of the patient. It is inappropriate to seek diagnostic truth to satisfy the interests of the practitioner, particularly if the benefits for the patient are only small or perhaps not even obvious. An investigation should be initiated only if it is likely to be of some benefit to the patient. If the possibility of benefit is unknown, then there is justification in considering the action, but if an investigation is required purely for interest, except for scientific study (which is a separate issue and will not be considered within this chapter), then it should not be suggested as an option.

It is important to recognize the tools used in the decision-making process. The practitioner should consider which decision-making processes the patient will utilize when assessing and evaluating their own situations. Efforts to maintain consistency in questioning should be considered. Be aware that innocuous changes in wording of questions, even during general conversation, can have powerful effects on patients and their responses.

In the information-gathering process, clinical signs and symptoms have to be considered in addition to social factors. Everyone should be approached as an individual; what is poor quality of life for one person may be an acceptable life for another. Some people do not want surgical intervention to prolong their life span, if the quality is going to be poor. Remember that any process or system is only as good as the information fed into it. The decision-maker must be able to justify the decisions made.

Decision-making is usually reinforced by experience and past knowledge, and this information must be collated in some systematic form. Interpretations of evidence rely on accurate judgements. However, if these judgements are questioned or examined at any time, then the practitioner must be able to justify the actions taken and this can best be supported by keeping accurate records of discussions.

It is difficult to judge how much information to give to patients and their families. Do we tell them what we think they ought to be told or what they want to know? Bear in mind also that the average patient knows very little about exactly how much they want to know. However, if we are serious about the patient's views, then we must ensure that they receive all of the relevant facts of the situation presented in a format that they can understand (see Chapter 7 for informed consent guidance).

When discussing options in healthcare, and possibly issues around risks and prognosis, the practitioner should be aware of cognitive illusion. This occurs when people are faced with the probability of survival rather than death, with surgery leading to survival. In such cases, the patient is more likely to choose surgery, as it is a more attractive option than death. At this stage then, the practitioner should be aware of local and national morbidity and mortality figures associated with the presenting disease and treatment options, otherwise values associated with the options cannot realistically be considered.

Diagnostic reasoning

While we all need some rigidity in the form of protocols that support quality and standard setting, there will be occasions when the protocol is not sufficient and clinical diagnostic reasoning will have to be applied. Diagnostic reasoning requires the processing of data according to the circumstance; in healthcare the problem-solving circumstance is often complex and multiple (Carnevali et al., 1984).

Clinical diagnostic reasoning requires an information-processing approach, considering the inputs/cues (symptoms and test results) and the outputs/options. It involves formulation of a clinical hypothesis following consideration of data, and then testing the hypothesis to allow decisions to be made. The practitioner requires a well-structured and organized knowledge base to allow information to be recalled and analysed whenever required. Clinicians do usually utilize similar strategies for information seeking in order to produce a diagnosis.

Initially patients are asked routine general questions such as:

- 'What made you go along to your GP?'
- 'How long have you had this problem?'
- 'Are these your only symptoms?'
- 'What illnesses have troubled your family?

When something significant is reported. the information-seeking questions become more specific, for example:

- 'Is the pain severe enough to keep you awake at night?'
- 'Is the pain worse after a meal?'
- 'Is the blood bright or dark red?'

Clinical reasoning is the thinking and decision-making processes associated with clinical practice, the process of hypothetical deductive reasoning. A clinical hypothesis is based on data collected, but it is the clinicians' knowledge base which is the key to success of the process (Grant and Marsden, 1987). The significance of dark red as opposed to bright red blood in colorectal bleeding has to be understood to make the response and future actions meaningful and appropriate. When making inferences to form hypotheses, the choice of relevant or irrelevant variables is vital; there is no value in considering inappropriate factors from the history or offering irrelevant options.

Clinical decision-making

Observe closely experienced clinicians in their information-seeking interview technique; certain patterns and themes will recur and prompt the direction of the interview and the diagnostic methods advocated. Experienced practitioners often rely on a systematic series of questions designed to supply a clinical picture that can be analysed in order to arrive at a well-reasoned decision. Of course, judgement is required to determine how much importance should be attached to detail given by the patient, and if their reporting skills can be trusted to be accurate. Consistency is required, particularly in cue finding and recommended actions, although we can never be sure that each practitioner will identify the level of importance of reported symptoms in the same manner.

Clinical decision-making can be complex and requires restructuring and reconsideration of the problem throughout the solving process to allow judgements to be logical and quantitative. Factors in the clinical judgement scenario include:

1 making a diagnosis
2 selecting a treatment route
3 evaluating outcomes
4 considering probabilities
5 assessing views and preferences (Eddy et al., 1983).

It is possible that individual reasoning can become fixed and it may become difficult to reformulate, with over-confidence also being a problem. Once a decision has been selected, it may be difficult to think of any other possible suitable solutions. Decision-making relies on a store of knowledge. However, information-processing capacity is inhibited by the amount of information that can be held in the short-term memory at one time, and the clarity and accessibility of information stored in the long-term memory (Newell and Simon, 1972). So it is important to consider the presenting clinical scenario more than once and to ensure that following diagnosis the treatment options remain the most appropriate, preferred and agreed by both the clinical team and the patient.

When faced with uncertainty, decision analysis decomposes a problem, allowing inspection of the attraction of each possible action (Doubilet and McNeil, 1988). However, you should be confident in the theory and science associated with evidence-based care and clinical effectiveness before embarking on the search for solutions. Clinical decision-making has to be supported by evidence in the first instance: controlled trials, quasi-experimental (epidemiological) studies, system-aided judgements and systematic reviews, as well as decision analysis programmes and peer-aided judgements (Dowie and Elstein, 1988).

Intuitive judgement

Analysis is seen as breaking things down in order to understand them better, while intuition leaves the problem in its original form. Unfortunately, analysis and intuition may not always bring about the same conclusion, which can lead to confusion or even conflict. Often the experience of the practitioner will determine whether they favour the intuitive or analytical approach; however, both approaches can be successfully used in conjunction. Often nurses, relying heavily on subjective data to recognize signs of early deterioration, are capable of recognizing when something is wrong without being able to identify why (Benner, 1984). The value of this skill should not be disregarded.

The cognitive continuum model of Kenneth Hammond et al. (1980) provides a theory as to how decisions are made, based on six modes of enquiry:

- intuitive judgement
- peer-aided judgement
- system-aided judgement
- quasi-experiment
- controlled trial
- scientific experiment.

All of these modes involve intuition or analysis to a greater or lesser extent. Usually the less well structured a task the more we need to rely on intuition to support our judgements. Well-structured tasks are analysed and poorly structured tasks are approached using intuition (Hammond et al., 1980).

A systematic approach

Collecting defined information in a systematic manner should identify high-risk groups, but thought and judgement should constantly be applied, looking for that extra piece of information that will contribute to the analysis of options and outcomes. Systems and models for information collection need to be consistent and relevant. When taking a history from the patient there should be a pattern or framework that complements the mode of enquiry.

The nursing process

A structured approach to problem solving could be supported by 'the nursing process', which follows the traditional model of assess, plan, implement and evaluate. Since the early 1980s, the concept of a systematic approach to problem solving in nursing has been advocated in the UK. This concept was previously identified in the US and concentrated on the provision of holistic and individual care. Unfortunately, although the nursing process is applied to most areas of clinical practice in the UK, it is essentially a care-planning paper exercise, which is poorly understood and often applied with unnecessary complexity. Perhaps now is a good time for nurses to re-evaluate their assessment and care-planning processes to ensure that they do complement and assist the delivery of care rather than hinder the development of rational, logical practitioners.

When faced with uncertainty

If there is certainty of a disease, then the experienced clinician will initiate treatment. If there is uncertainty within the range of 10–90 per cent, further investigations are likely to be pursued. However, if the clinician is fairly certain that there is no case to treat, then he or she will temporize (Spielgelhalter, 1985). Of course, the door must always be open. Instruct the patient that there are no obvious causes for the symptoms, nothing obvious to worry about at this stage, but if symptoms are exacerbated then further investigation may be required and can be initiated.

It can be argued that a better decision may be achieved with an attempted structured decision analysis than from trusting intuition. However, the value of prediction and the need to acknowledge uncertainty cannot be overlooked. Uncertainty will be influenced as facts are gathered; then a process of weighting the evidence can result in a prediction. Prognostic and risk indices or diagnostic scoring systems assist in this process. In the area of gastroenterology, many scoring systems have been considered, some based on statistical logistical regression and some quite simply adding up the number of positive symptoms (Spiegelhalter, 1985). Obviously, if a situation is random, then a predictable, systematic approach cannot be applied.

During the decision-making process a set of plausible, reasonable solutions will be considered. Of course, as probability is a subjective assessment of something happening, the expert can make an assessment and consider the probability of reasonable likelihood, more quickly, more efficiently and more accurately than the novice, as the ability to predict with accuracy is enhanced with knowledge

Good probability assessments come from individuals who are aware of what they know and do not know. It is important to remember that tests and investigations may not all be sufficiently sensitive to pick up the disease, therefore the practitioner should be aware of the validity and reliability of the test. When detecting colorectal cancer, for example, there is a variety of diagnostic tests that can be chosen. Often the choice of procedure depends on who is to perform it, the circumstances of the presentation and the circumstances of the patient. The problem then is to decide which test is appropriate. When faced with options and uncertainties it is best to do what the majority of others are doing and to be guided by senior colleagues and professional bodies. The practitioner is less likely to be sued for requesting too much information than too little at the time of investigation (Eddy, 1988). However, a defensive approach to diagnosis is wasteful and unnecessary.

Decision-making frameworks

A variety of decision-making frameworks can be utilized to help increase clarity of thought and provide a diagrammatic illustration for the patient. A small number of those regularly used in healthcare are listed below.

Cognitive mapping exercises

A cognitive map requires production of visual representation, retrieved from the knowledge store. It is usually in the form of a diagram or chart indicating interconnected ideas. Patients cannot draw on such an extensive knowledge store for their information processing when faced with decisions and therefore have to rely on the data supplied by the practitioner.

Statistical decision theory

Utilizing a decision-making framework should result in the best decision being made for the individual concerned. Statistical decision theory considers how decisions can be made using an analytical approach.

In the first instance, there needs to be agreement that there is a decision to be made, and that there are appropriate options available. Sometimes people prefer to accept the first reasonable option rather than looking for the best one. Therefore there must be agreement about the need to look for a decision and the options. Decision theory requires calculation of probabilities and values to produce decisions that will benefit the patient (McGuire, 1985). Some people are happy to relinquish their right to have a preference, choosing to leave the decision to the expert, as sometimes the burden of being forced to look at choices can have severe psychological consequences (McNeil and Pauker, 1979).

Statistical decision theory requires a mathematical approach to the choice of actions. Each action has an outcome and each outcome is assigned a probability value. This decision-making approach is particularly useful when there is risk associated with the outcomes, as the risks can easily be displayed in percentage values from local or national statistics. Whenever statistical information is available it should be used in preference to estimates of probability.

Decision trees

Similar to cognitive mapping exercises, decision trees should illustrate the problem and solutions in a structured way, clearly showing available outcomes and choices. This approach utilizes branches on a tree to attach each available option and possible consequence, clearly illustrating the available outcomes and choices. Professional expertise and knowledge is necessary to ensure that all options are included on the tree. Values are given to each option or outcome and the option with the biggest value is considered the best available option. This is clearly not a method that can be utilized when time is short, for example in a resuscitation situation. It would be expected that the practitioner already has a quick analytical model available for decision-making in the emergency situation.

It is possible that different people will attach different values to available options; therefore it is important that all members of the healthcare team have some common values. Different figures may still be attached to options, but this is acceptable providing the process can be evaluated and is to be expected if the patient is considered as an individual in the process. It is possible to be biased, and influence outcomes by the values attached. Personal beliefs and preferences may influence predictions and forecasts. The only way to address this problem is to be aware of it. When attaching options to decision trees, remember that the option of choosing to do nothing should be included. The important factor to remember when assigning values or discussing probabilities is to capture the personal preferences and values of the patient. The decision analysis should be capable of showing personal feelings and meanings.

Whichever method is utilized in discussions and decision-making, the practitioner must ensure that all options considered are appropriate and justifiable. The availability of time and resources will always be a major restrictor, and therefore a vital consideration in the decision-making process. Occasionally, it may not be appropriate to consider all possible options; they may be too traumatic, expensive or unethical.

Cost/benefit analysis

When deciding on the management of patients, the cost of resources has to be taken into account. Often a sequence of decisions is required by a variety of people, many of whom will apply a different analysis of available options and outcomes; this can be confusing for the patient and frustrating for other clinicians.

When considering quantity and quality, we should not only look at cost-effective analysis, but also at cost/benefit analysis. Rather than choosing the cheapest way to achieve an outcome, we should consider the most beneficial way of accessing options. When looking at costs do not confuse accounting boundaries (internal restrictions) with economic ones that belong to society in general.

Analysis and critique of conceptual frameworks

With the introduction of care pathways and algorithms, we need to consider if judgements of the type required in the hospital environment are simple enough to fit into a framework or algorithm. If all clinical decisions are supported by an analytical approach, is there a place for intuition?

Knowledge of rules and procedures is unquestionably a basic requirement. However, procedural knowledge and prepositional knowledge are different. You may know how to do something, but during the procedure, prepositional skills are required. Experts know when a change of plan or alternative course is required; their practical clinical skills allow them to make the necessary changes. The argument against direct acceptance of care pathways is that they may reduce the ability of the individual to make analytical decisions when faced with uncertainty, or that when prepositional skills are required the practitioner will not have these appropriately developed. The author acknowledges that nurses in particular must work within algorithms and care pathways. However, it is always worth considering the presenting situation to ensure that, after careful thought and analysis, the route advised in the pathway seems to be the most appropriate for the individual circumstance. Also remember that, at times, a rational and scientific approach to problem solving may not be appropriate; intuition cannot always be weighted but should not be disregarded.

The evidence-based approach

Practising evidence-based care requires a firm grasp of available information. The opportunity for systematic appraisal of the recent published literature may be limited due to clinical time restraints. Textbooks are often relied on for valuable information, but due to publishing delays and the vast speed of developments in healthcare, they are often out of date by the time they are printed. Therefore, it may be difficult to acquire data, let alone have time to appraise them. However, lack of time to keep up to date is not a valid excuse for the advanced nurse practitioner, who must be aware of developments in healthcare.

The scientific papers will guide decision-making, identifying available care options, but applicability of a recommendation to your own area of practice requires specific knowledge and experience. Clinical experience is invaluable. Knowing when to take action is a skill that is learnt over time.

Many situations reported in the literature are rare, and you should remember this, as it will help when considering them in relation to probability assessment. The normal routine occurrence is under-reported, so the inexperienced practitioner may find misrepresentation in medical and nursing texts and journals. Remember that symptoms may be from a number of diseases. If the pattern appears unfamiliar, this may be because a multiple diagnosis is required.

Experience versus education

When clinical decision-making skills taught by exposure to academic processes are combined with years of experience, information searching and analytical and evaluative skills are enhanced (Girot, 2000). Teaching strategies should develop independent learning and support development of a knowledge base that is well organized, allowing interrelated information to be considered (Terry and Higgs, 1993). In a study evaluating the influence of academic study on the development of critical thinking and its application to clinical practice, nurses exposed to advanced study were found to have significantly better clinical decision-making skills than non-academic nurses (Girot, 2000).

Reflection

There will always be someone who suggests that had they been in your situation, they would have approached it differently, but of course they were not party to all of the facts supporting your decision. Therefore, the rule is that decisions and value attachments must be justifiable at the time of the analysis. Hindsight and retrospective analysis are, however, useful for learning, and can be incorporated into structured learning as part of clinical supervision. Analysis of a past action as described by Schon (1987) is valuable, as it can be applied even in a new environment or in cases of uncertainty. Reflection in action is not easy (Terry and Higgs, 1993), and audit can be very valuable for reflective analysis of action. Evaluation should always use a systematic approach.

As practice becomes more spontaneous and the practitioner more experienced, the opportunity for thinking about actions may be lost; therefore the advanced practitioner should utilize both clinical audit and regular reflection. The process of reflection has, at times, been misrepresented and inappropriately utilized. However, boredom or burn-out leading to rigid and restrictive practice can be reversed with reflection and/or clinical audit.

Ethical and moral considerations

Ethics is involved in any decision over actions. Our moral duty has got to be to create an environment and develop policies that respect important values. Ethical frameworks do not, however, solve the problem, but they do help to clarify and identify personal beliefs.

Conclusion

If we are ever going to be able to consider the patients' views, we must strive to ensure that they receive all of the relevant facts of the situation. However, consideration must be given to the volume of information that patients want to be given and to their ability to apply balance and logic when faced with stressful decisions, often while suffering from ill health. This chapter has identified some important principles for consideration in clinical decision-making; however it is not an academic process and experience will always aid judgements. Therefore, never be afraid to seek advice when faced with difficult decisions and do consider the power of reflection, both on action and in action.

References

Bandman E, Bandman B (1988) Critical Thinking in Nursing. Norwalk: Appleton and Lange.

Benner P (1984) From Novice to Expert: excellence and power in clinical nursing practice. Reading, Mass: Addison-Wesley.

Carnevali D, Mitchell P, Woods N, Tanner C (1984) Diagnostic Reasoning in Nursing. Philadelphia, Pa: Lippincott.

Doubilet P, McNeil BJ (1988) In: Dowie J, Elstein A (eds) Professional Judgment: a reader in clinical decision making. Cambridge: Cambridge University Press.

Dowie J, Elstein A (1988) Professional Judgment: a reader in clinical decision making. Cambridge: Cambridge University Press.

Eddy DM (1988) Variations in physician practice: the role of uncertainty. In: Dowie J, Elstein A (eds) Professional Judgment: a reader in clinical decision making. Cambridge: Cambridge University Press.

Eddy DM, Sanders LE, Eddy JF (1983) The value of screening for glaucoma with tonometry. Survey of Ophthalmology 28(3), 194–205.

Elstein AS, Shulman LS, Sprafka SA (1978) Medical Problem Solving: an analysis of clinical reasoning. Cambridge, Mass: Harvard University Press.

Eraker SA, Politser P (1982) How decisions are reached: physician and patient. Annals of Internal Medicine 97(2), 262–268.

Eraker SA, Sox HC (1981) Assessment of patients' preferences for therapeutic outcomes. Medical Decision Making 1, 29–39.

Gambrill E (1990) Critical Thinking in Clinical Practice. Oxford: Jossey-Bass.

Girot EA (2000) Graduate nurses: critical thinkers or better decision makers? Journal of Advanced Nursing 31(2), 288–297.

Grant J, Marsden P (1987) The structure of memorised knowledge in students and clinicians: an explanation for diagnostic expertise. Medical Education 21, 92–98.

Hammond K, McClelland GH, Mumpower J (1980) Human Judgment and Decision Making. New York: Hemisphere.

Jones SA, Brown L (1991) Critical thinking: impact of nursing education. Journal of Advanced Nursing 16, 529–533.

McGuire CH (1985) Medical problem solving: a critique of the literature. Journal of Medical Education 60, 587–595.

McNeil BJ, Pauker SG (1979) The patient's role in assessing the value of diagnostic tests. Radiology 132(3), 605–610.

Newell A, Simon HA (1972) Human Problem Solving. Englewood Cliffs, NJ: Prentice Hall.

Schon DA (1987) Educating the Reflective Practitioner. San Francisco, Calif: Jossey-Bass.

Spiegelhalter DJ (1985) Statistical methodology for evaluating gastrointestinal symptoms. Clinics in Gastroenterology 14(3), 489–515.

Terry W, Higgs J (1993) Educational programmes to develop clinical reasoning skills. Australian Journal of Physiotherapy 39(1), 47–51.

Watson G, Glaser WM (1991) Watson-Glaser Critical Thinking Appraisal Manual. New York: The Psychological Corporation, Harcourt Brace Jovanovich.

Further reading

Damian D, Tattersall MHN (1991) Letters to patients: improving communication in cancer care. Lancet 338, 923–925.

Degner LF, Sloan JA (1992) Decision making during serious illness: what role do patients really want to play? Journal of Clinical Epidemiology 45, 941–950.

CHAPTER 11

Clinical supervision

SURRINDER KAUR

Introduction

Clinical supervision was identified as a national initiative through the strategy *A Vision for the Future* (NHSME, 1993). Target 10 of the strategy advocated further exploration of the concept of clinical supervision and its application. One of the triggers that led to this was the concern arising from the Allitt Inquiry in 1991, which highlighted the need for nurses to receive support within their day-to-day practice, and argued that clinical supervision could actually assist in sustaining safe standards of clinical practice.

The purpose of this chapter is to:

• define clinical supervision
• identify the benefits of clinical supervision
• outline the models of clinical supervision
• briefly describe the processes and skills utilized in clinical supervision.

There are many definitions of clinical supervision; a common one is 'an exchange between practising professionals to enable the development of professional skills' (Butterworth and Faugier, 1992). In 1996, the UKCC issued a position statement in which the purpose of clinical supervision was stated as 'bringing practitioners and skilled supervisors together to reflect on practice. Supervision aims to identify solutions to problems pre-practice, and increase understanding of professional issues'. Further illumination occurs via the 1994 King's Fund executive summary on clinical supervision, which stated that clinical supervision was 'formal arrangements that enable nurses, midwives and health visitors to discuss their work regularly with other experienced professionals.... Clinical supervision involves reflection on practice in order to learn from experience and improve competence. An important part of the supervisor's role is to facilitate reflection and a learning process'.

Exercise

Briefly write down what the term 'clinical supervision' conjures up for you. Think about:

- what it means to you
- what are your fears about it?
- what would you ideally expect to gain from the process?

For the nurse practitioner who is developing a new role, the issue of clinical supervision is of paramount importance. First, to develop new knowledge and its application, second, to manage the emotional aspects of the role, and third, to develop the standards of clinical practice. Proctor (1987) identifies three functions of clinical supervision:

- formative
- restorative
- normative.

The formative function of clinical supervision is the educative function. Within this process, the supervisee (the person receiving supervision) will be able to articulate the relationship of the theory to practice in a critical way, identifying her own strengths, weaknesses and abilities, and gaining knowledge.

The restorative function of clinical supervision alludes to being supportive. Within this aspect, the supervisee's emotional responses and distress arising from stressful situations and relationships can be explored. The supportive environment gives the supervisee an opportunity to articulate her feelings and be listened to and valued, and to explore various coping strategies to manage her feelings and stresses.

The normative function of clinical supervision explores the managerial aspects of practice and the maintenance and development of standards. In practice, the supervisee is able to explore the departmental and organizational objectives and meet the standards of competence required. The implementation of evidence-based practice can be explored and supported within the context of change management.

Clinical supervision requires a balance of all three functions. The nurse practitioner needs to recognize that one function may predominate at particular times, according to individual needs. Equally, the nurse practitioner may find that these three functions cannot be explored with one supervisor and may actually require supervision on a one-to-one basis with a number of different supervisors based within and outside the organization.

Questions that may arise include:

- How will the nurse practitioner/specialist obtain supervision?
- Who is the best person to provide that supervision?
- As the only nurse practitioner/specialist within that speciality, is supervision obtained from a member of the medical profession?
- Is it possible to set up supervision across geographical and organizational boundaries?
- Is it possible to have some forms of supervision from other non-gastroentrology healthcare professionals?

Case study

I have only just got into post as a nurse consultant and there is no one in a similar post in my trust at present. Fortunately I have an established network of people I have used for a number of years to obtain supervision. In order to develop the teaching aspects of my role, I have an educational supervisor based in the university, who is really supporting me to explore and develop this aspect in my new role. I use a general manager as a supervisor to help me look at how I can manage change within the department and organizationally; he is very good at enabling me to look at my leadership style and manage the politics within the department and in the trust. As a non-nurse, the general manger really challenges me and has enabled me to reframe my thinking on many issues. I use the deputy director of nursing for personal supervision in relation to my career development and to discuss the tensions that I am feeling in my new role as I struggle to define and develop it. My biggest concern at present is that there is not another nurse who has more advanced knowledge of my sphere of practice in the trust; I really need to discuss the technical details of my clinical practice with someone who works in the field. I have discussed this with the medical consultant on the unit. He helped set up my post and we work closely together developing the clinical guidelines and protocols that I shall need to support my practice. The medical consultant's style is quite directive, he likes to say what needs to be done. So I have had to spend some time explaining to him what clinical supervision is and the facilitative style I want him to provide! I have given him some literature to read on it and because he wants the post to be successful and to be supportive, he has been responsive, taking his role as clinical supervisor seriously. I have even managed to persuade him to go to a workshop on clinical supervision to prepare him for the role.

The benefits of clinical supervision

Professional development benefits

The nurse practitioner, utilizing reflection and documenting clinical supervision sessions, can ensure that this becomes part of fulfilling her post-registration educational practice requirements (UKCC, 1992) to show evidence of ongoing learning as well as evidence of ongoing personal practice development. Documented evidence can later be used to accredit experiential learning if there is a desire to study at a higher degree level.

By capturing the learning taking place within clinical supervision, there is a clear link with lifelong learning and the clinical governance agenda. Clinical supervision will also enable the nurse practitioner to manage the stresses felt within her new role and the stress that may be associated with moving and developing new practices. Clinical supervision is beneficial not only for professional stress, but also to assist the development of personal coping strategies. The nurse practitioner will be involved in developing practice within a wide clinical area and therefore clinical supervision will provide an arena to address some of these issues, both by receiving clinical supervision and giving clinical supervision to others.

Clinical supervision should ultimately have a direct beneficial link to patient care, providing a safe, supportive environment for individuals or groups of nurses/medical staff to come together in a constructive professional manner. By examining clinical practice, both the individual and the public can be assured of protection through safe practice and rising standards.

Ultimately, clinical supervision should also be beneficial to the organization by its contribution to the clinical governance framework and through longer-term contributions to reducing staff sickness, staff recruitment and retention problems.

Models of clinical supervision

The nurse practitioner can access a variety of clinical supervision models. The models include:

- one-to-one supervision
- group supervision
- network supervision.

Within each model the individual can choose the supervisor from:

* the same profession
* another profession
* a similar grade
* a higher grade
* based in the same organization
* based in another organization.

In the first instance, the nurse practitioner would be expected to identify with her manager the best mechanism to access supervision. The factors that will influence choice will relate to:

* the trust's strategy for clinical supervision
* the availability of skilled supervisors
* personal time and diary commitments
* personal needs required from clinical supervision.

Ownership of the clinical supervision model is an essential factor in its success. The nurse practitioner needs to identify the purpose of the clinical supervision, the strengths, weaknesses and resource implications personally and for the gastroentrology department and the organization, in order to determine the feasibility of implementing a particular model.

Exercise

Considering each model of supervision, list the advantages and disadvantages to you personally of choosing that particular model, utilizing the headings as identified in Table 11.1.

One-to-one supervision

The previous case study describes the model of supervision set up to obtain expert supervision in relation to aspects of an educational, managerial and clinical role, as well as personal career development needs. This is on a one-to-one basis, using a variety of people from different disciplines and different seniority from both within and outside the organization.

In the first instance, the nurse practitioner may require clinical supervision with an expert in order to explore the specific detailed competencies and knowledge required for specialized practice. It may be that there is no other expert in this specialist area of nursing in the

Table 11.1 Choosing a model of supervision

Model of supervision	Advantages	Disadvantages	Best option identified
One-to-one supervision: • With someone from the same profession • With someone from another profession • With someone of same grade • With someone of higher grade • In the organization • Outside of the organization			
Group supervision • With people from the same profession • With people from another profession • With people of same grade • With people of higher grade			
Network supervision • In the organization • Outside of the organization			

organization. This means that the nurse practitioner may need to access someone from another organization, which can lead to problems in terms of diary commitments and travel, although telephone/ teleconferencing clinical supervision would be an option to explore. Equally, it may be necessary in the first instance to receive this form of clinical supervision from a medical colleague. This in itself requires detailed setting up of the model, as clinical supervision may mean something entirely different within the medical field. Therefore, training for the medical and nursing staff to give and receive clinical supervision should actually take place together. There may be aspects of clinical supervision that the nurse practitioner is able to explore with other nurse practitioners, consultant nurses or clinical nurse specialists from a different clinical speciality on a one-to-one level within the organization. And there may be common issues in setting up a new role that can be explored on a one-to-one basis.

Group supervision

Group supervision can also be developed as a model. The group could consist of other like-minded gastroenterology nurses and a mixture of clinical nurse specialist and consultant nurses from a variety of disciplines within the organization. Alternatively, group supervision could be confined to nursing, medical and therapy staff from the gastroenterological field.

Network supervision

It may be that the gastroenterology nurse practitioners actually develop a network supervision model in which they meet together to discuss practice with a variety of people. They may actually choose to use all three models at different times or even simultaneously, at times during the course of their practice.

Reflective learning

The critical basis of clinical supervision is the ability to reflect on everyday activities and to learn from these. Kolb's (1984) cycle of learning from experience, as illustrated in Figure 11.1, is probably familiar to most people.

Boud et al. (1985) highlighted the cyclical nature of reflection. The nurse practitioner can go through this cycle a number of times before she recognizes the commitment to action required. It is acceptable to return to the same experience and reflect on it from new perspectives a number of times to tease out the learning and to continue to understand the practice. Reflection is a critical skill for the nurse practitioner, starting with thinking about an experience, then analysing and evaluating it. Reflecting on practice will enable the nurse practitioner to:

- gain insight and understanding
- identify further learning needs
- identify the learning from the experience and its application to future practice
- explore the strengths and weaknesses of people, situations and practice
- identify a plan for personal and practice development
- improve critical questioning abilities
- reframe situations, feelings and attitudes
- solve problems
- develop a framework in which to act more effectively as a role model.

Reflection can take place in a number of ways. Schon (1987) identified two types of reflection. First is 'reflection in action', in which the reflection takes place as the experience is occurring during clinical practice. This reflection will influence the decisions the nurse makes and the care given in the immediate situation. 'Reflection on action' is retrospective in that it looks back on incidents that have occurred and the process is undertaken through discussion or by writing or drawing them.

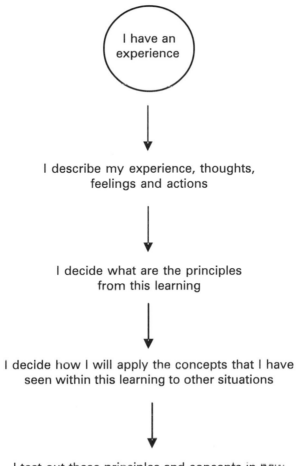

Figure 11.1 Learning from experiences (Kolb, 1984).

When undertaking retrospective reflection, it is important to have a framework within which to structure it. A simple framework is to ask:

- Why was a particular incident important to me?
- How do I feel about it?
- What was disappointing about the incident?
- What could have been done differently within the incident?
- What actions would I take in the future if a similar situation arose?
- What have I learnt through this experience?

When writing or talking in a reflective process it is important that the nurse makes 'I' statements and does not fall into the trap of being defensive to justify a course of actions. During reflection it is acceptable for the nurse practitioner to say how they really feel, even if it may be uncomfortable or 'politically incorrect'.

The process of beginning to reflect can be difficult, therefore trigger phrases can be used as a start, for example:

- I felt good when…
- I felt angry when…
- I felt hurt when…
- My beliefs about this are…
- My values about this are…
- My prejudices are…
- Alternative options I would consider are…
- Contributing factors that made this good were…
- The contributing factors that made this difficult situation were…
- I would handle things differently by…
- What would happen if…?

Exercise

Using the above framework or the triggers, write about or discuss with a colleague a recent clinical event or experience.

Reflection through drawing

Drawing it can help personal reflection prior to a clinical supervision session; indeed, it is a helpful technique if the supervisee has difficulty in expressing an issue during a session. Reflective drawing is not about being an artist; matchstick men and/or symbols can be used to represent a situation. By explaining what the drawing represents, the process of reflection begins.

Exercise

- Draw a situation that has happened in your clinical practice.
- Now draw how you would ideally like the situation to look in the future.

- By comparing the two drawings and discussing them, id
  situation arose as it did, what you have learnt from it
  would work towards creating your ideal situation.

The role and responsibilities of the supervisee

The supervisee is responsible for ensuring that the clinical supervisor selected has the appropriate level of skills to facilitate his or her supervision needs. Supervisors should be chosen on the basis of:

- their ability to share their expertise, skills, knowledge and experience
- the quality of their communication and facilitation skills
- their ability to critically question and challenge
- their ability to assist new perspectives and mental pictures to be developed.

The supervisor and supervisee, in identifying the role and responsibilities of each, should develop an oral or written contract. The role of the nurse practitioner in receiving clinical supervision is to ensure that the session has been prepared for in terms of identifying the issues and experiences that will be explored with the clinical supervisor. In the NHS, everyone has time constraints, therefore it is the responsibility of the supervisee to arrive at sessions on time and to keep to time within the sessions. The supervisee is responsible for keeping her personal records of clinical supervision sessions and reflecting on the issues raised. As a supervisee, the nurse practitioner has the right to receive clinical supervision in a non-judgemental manner and to expect the clinical supervisor to maintain confidentiality. However, the supervisee must also maintain confidentiality and accountability in relation to patients and colleagues. The supervisee is responsible for participating in the session in a sensitive manner, respecting both the clinical supervisor and other members of the group, if they are participating in group supervision.

The skills that the gastroenterology nurse will require to receive clinical supervision are many, but essentially they are:

- listening skills
- assertiveness
- respect
- reflection skills
- decision-making skills
- assessment planning
- evaluation skills.

The role and responsibility of the nurse practitioner as a supervisor

The nurse practitioner not only needs to be able to receive clinical supervision to enhance clinical practice, but will also be expected to be a clinical supervisor giving supervision to other nurses and medical staff.

As a supervisor, the nurse practitioner will be responsible for starting and finishing clinical supervision sessions on time, and for minimizing the number of interruptions during sessions. The clinical supervisor will be responsible for managing the supervisee and maintaining the focus of the discussion. Ensuring that a safe and comfortable environment is created for the supervisee is important to facilitate good discussion. The supervisee will need skilled support to explore issues and reach her own decisions and conclusions, and she should keep a record of the overall summary of each supervision session. Documentation of the session needs to be agreed by both parties in the first instance. It is important that both parties maintain the ground rules of the time, frequency, record keeping and confidentiality of clinical supervision sessions, ensuring that there are clearly established rules and responsibilities understood by both the supervisor and supervisee.

Skills the gastroenterology nurse will require as a clinical supervisor are:

- organizational
- listening
- assertiveness
- managing conflict
- facilitation
- reflection
- decision-making
- summarizing
- paraphrasing
- reflecting back
- non-judgemental communication skills
- open body language.

Clinical supervisors needing supervision

The nurse practitioner, if she is acting as a supervisor for the first time, will be practising by transferring skills used from other situations into a unique situation. Often clinical supervisors themselves will require support and supervision on their supervisory skills development. This may be provided by the organization, which is rolling out clinical supervision models across the whole organization, and therefore the nurse practitioner needs to be able to participate within this. It is equally important for the nurse practitioner as a clinical leader to influence the development of clinical supervision within the policy and strategic context of her organization. This can be done through contribution to the professional and practice development forums within the organization.

Evaluating clinical supervision

It is important to evaluate the effectiveness of clinical supervision. This needs to take place both on an individual level and with the clinical supervisor. The purpose of evaluation is to provide insight into whether the clinical supervision sessions have met the intended aims and needs of those involved, and to identify how the processes of clinical supervision can be developed and enhanced further. Additionally, the overall impact of the clinical supervision on both the individual and her practice needs to be examined.

At its simplest level, evaluation can be a nurse practitioner looking back on the clinical supervision sessions and asking:

• Did I carry out the actions agreed at clinical supervision sessions?
• Can I identify three changes in my personal practice as a consequence of clinical supervision?
• Can I identify three changes in ideas, attitudes or values I previously held?
• What changes in me and my personal practice have other people noticed and fed back to me?
• Am I managing my workload more effectively?
• Am I managing myself and the way I feel differently?

Other questions that can be asked during evaluation are related to the sessions themselves, for example whether the nurse attended all the clinical supervision sessions and punctually, and whether she prepared for the sessions. In evaluating the sessions, it is also important to provide feedback to the clinical supervisor on whether the style and content of the supervision sessions have met the personal needs.

The clinical supervisor would need to evaluate whether the caseload of supervisees was adequate to manage, and whether there had been adequate supervision of the clinical supervisees. The clinical supervisor needs to evaluate whether overall the patients have received a better standard of care as a result of nurse supervision. To evaluate this can be quite difficult, and clinical supervision needs to be given time before results can be seen. Evaluation can take place by examining complaints records and clinical supervision records, or through interviews, observation and questionnaires.

Training for clinical supervision

In an ideal world it would be useful for all staff working within gastroenterology to have received clinical supervision training together. This would enable a variety of clinical supervision models to be used in an area and would support nursing, medical and therapy practitioners in giving and receiving clinical supervision on a multiprofessional basis.

Training does not have to be difficult to be organized. There is a wealth of open and distance learning materials that groups can work through, and facilitators can be brought in to assist the unit in developing its own philosophy and stance in the implementation of clinical supervision. Good clinical supervision within the gastroenterology unit can enhance the development of teamwork.

Conclusion

Clinical supervision is a critical support mechanism for all professionals engaged in direct patient care. It serves to increase learning to ensure standards of care are consistently maintained and developed. In a busy world, it provides a safe haven for practitioners to be listened to and respected as individuals who have the desire to work at their maximum potential.

References

Allitt Inquiry (1991) Independent enquiry relating to deaths on the children's ward at Grantham and Kesteven General Hospital during the period February to April 1991. London: HSMO.

Boud D, Keogh R, Walker D (1985) Reflection: turning experience into learning. London: Kogan Page.

Butterworth T, Faugier J (1992) Clinical supervision in nursing, midwifery and health visiting, a briefing paper. Manchester: University of Manchester.

King's Fund (1994) Clinical Supervision – an Executive Summary. London: Nursing Development Units, King's Fund.

Kolb DA (1984) Experiential Learning. New Jersey: Prentice Hall.

NHS Management Executive (1993) A Vision for the Future. London: NHSME.

Proctor B (1987) Supervision; a co-operative exercise in accountability. In: Marken M, Payne M (eds) Enabling and Enduring. Leicester: National Youth Bureau/Council for Education and Training in Youth and Community Work.

Schon DA (1987) Educating the Reflective Practitioner. San Francisco, Calif: Jossey Bass.

United Kingdom Central Council for Nursing, Midwifery and Health Visiting (1992) Post Registration Education Practice. London: UKCC.

United Kingdom Central Council for Nursing, Midwifery and Health Visiting (1996) Position Statement on Clinical Supervision for Nursing and Health Visiting. London: UKCC.

Further reading

Field A, Roswell V, Dolan B, Kaur S (1998) Clinical Super ...vision, a Workbook. Part of the the West Midlands Collaborative Clinical Supervision Project. NHS Executive.

Open University (1998) Clinical Supervision, a Development Pack for Nurses. The Open University.

CHAPTER 12

Reflecting on practice and portfolio development

ALDINE ALSOP

Introduction

This chapter explores the concept of reflection as a basis for professional work and as a process through which practitioners can continue to develop their skills and their understanding of practice. It will set the notion of reflection into the wider context of advanced nursing practice. Acquiring the ability to learn from experience and to generate knowledge should enable nurses to develop their capacity for effective practice. Enhancing nurses' ability to define and solve problems, to develop reasoning skills and to be critically aware of their practice should strengthen their position as advanced practitioners. This chapter will show how insights emerging from reflective processes might be logged in portfolio form to show evidence of continuing professional development.

Skills for complex practice

Nurses, like all other healthcare professionals today, are practising in a complex world of health and social care. The context of care delivery is marked by instability and change that requires nurses to adopt practices that not only work effectively, but that also maintain the growth and development of the profession (Batehup, 1994). As Palmer (1994) pointed out, nurses are also facing an increasing obligation to evaluate and improve practice. So not only are nurses required to take steps to maintain the quality and effectiveness of their practice in a constantly changing environment, they are also expected to develop their practice to a higher level of proficiency for the benefit of the profession and those it serves.

174

Nursing practice has been described as dynamic, constantly changing, frustrating, challenging and exciting, all at the same time (Bulman, 1994 p131), but integral to that is the continuing requirement to treat people as individuals and in a flexible and responsive way. To this end, nurses would seem to need well-developed reasoning skills to assist them in understanding and resolving the complex patient problems encountered in practice (Fonteyn, 1995). Learning to appraise practice critically and knowing what steps to take to refine practice should enable nurses to develop new levels of competence. Developing the ability to practise reflectively may be one way of addressing these challenges and achieving these goals.

Advancing practice through reflection

Boud et al. (1993 p9) described reflection as 'those processes in which learners engage to recapture, notice and re-evaluate their experiences, to work with the experience and turn it into learning'. The process of reflection involves a series of mental activities that help to determine what has emerged during an experience and what was learned from it. Revisiting the experience in our mind, taking note of key features of the event, exploring for ourselves what happened and what the consequences were, and establishing how this adds to, or changes, what we already know, is the essence of reflection (Alsop, 2000). Only by reviewing situations can insight be gained into the effectiveness of current practice so that sensible judgements can be made in the future.

Palmer et al. (1994) considered reflection to be the retrospective contemplation of practice, suggesting that a careful review had to take place of what had happened previously. The review must involve analysing and interpreting the information recalled. This process should reveal the knowledge used in the situation and what other knowledge might have been helpful, and it should prompt the practitioner to speculate on how a situation might have been handled differently. Reflection, therefore, should encourage an individual to search for knowledge that helps to fill the gap, so that it can be stored for future reference. It should also help practitioners to identify how they can make modifications to practice in the light of new experience, knowledge and insights, and so improve their practice. As Hull and Redfern (1996, p92) concluded, reflection is about thinking, learning from experience and making use of that learning in the future.

The art of practice

Donald Schon (1983, 1987) popularized the notion of reflective practice by exposing and attempting to describe how professionals behave and by suggesting how they might learn to operate differently by reflecting on their practice. Hull and Redfern (1996) pointed out that Schon was not proposing anything new, he was merely trying to help practitioners to make sense of their practice and to develop new levels of understanding that would lead to changes and improvements in the way they work. Reflective practice was proposed as a way of dealing with the difficulty experienced by practitioners, of trying to solve problems using predefined solutions in situations where unique and complex problems prevailed. Such solutions were unlikely to prove effective as they did not take into account the varying needs and circumstances of individual service users. The complexity of practice, its uncertainty, instability and uniqueness could not be accommodated through technical rationality that tended to set common procedures for everything. An alternative way of approaching practice was required. Schon suggested that practitioners needed to become professional artists who could adopt an approach to problem solving that allowed creative, novel solutions to be explored. Sometimes practitioners needed to modify what they were doing and adapt to find ways of doing things that were outside of their current experience. This would demand not only the ability to reflect on actions that had already taken place but also the capacity to reflect in action, in order to modify practice in progress.

Reflecting in action (often referred to as 'thinking on one's feet') involves being alert to changing circumstances as they occur, revising decisions and taking a new course of action in light of new information. Practitioners who reflect in action can thus make reasoned decisions to modify intervention and accommodate change if the need arises, and therefore make a difference to the outcome. Reflection *on* action, on the other hand, entails thinking back over an event that has already finished. The learning that arises can make a difference only to future practice and future situations. Reflection in action prompts changes to be made while dealing with the situation, so that the outcome is the best that can be achieved at the time. Some situations will thus demand a quick, urgent response and a change to the intervention currently being implemented. In other situations, a practitioner may have longer to consider what other action could be taken that will make a difference. Reflecting on an incident after the event should highlight strengths and deficiencies in the way in which problems were addressed and should help to consolidate the learning that occurred overall.

Reflective practice is thus perceived as a process that not only enables practitioners to deal effectively with the immediacy of care of individuals, but also helps practitioners to gain a real understanding of practice, to bring about improvements in their own practice and to change nursing practice for the future. Engaging consciously and conscientiously in reflection should therefore assist advanced practitioners not only to develop their own professional practice but also to contribute to the development of the nursing profession as a whole.

Eraut (1994) held a view that much of what an expert practitioner actually does is, in fact, ongoing and non-reflective because it falls into the category of unproblematic, everyday practice. Practitioners just implement what works. It is only when situations are not normal and are in need of special attention that reflective processes are triggered. The actual trigger might be an unexpected action or outcome, or just an intuitive feeling of unease that something is not quite right. The processes of framing the problem (problem setting) and of identifying possible solutions will be that much more deliberate. It would seem that the greater the level of a nurse's expertise, the greater the amount of that nurse's work that might fall into the 'unproblematic' category. However, this does not account for changes that have to be accommodated because of changing external factors as opposed to just changes in actual practice. In some respects, however, it could also be argued that deciding what has been encountered before, and what is to be considered as needing special attention, is also a reflective practice. The practitioner has to judge whether his or her existing knowledge can be used effectively in the new situation.

L'Aiguille (1994), on the other hand, argued that reflection also prevents practitioners from becoming complacent with everyday aspects of work. It provides a means of untangling different aspects of a problem, situation or incident to learn why it occurred and how it might have been different. It can help in developing an understanding of complex interpersonal and interprofessional situations. While highlighting behaviour that is unhelpful to a situation, reflection can also help to identify skills, qualities and strengths that produce effective results. Vital lessons can thus be learned about the meaning of nursing practice and about the contribution that nurses make to patient care that will be of benefit to the nursing profession (L'Aiguille, 1994).

Brookfield (1995) took the arguments further to suggest that practising critical reflection should mean being serious about examining one's own theoretical assumptions and practices. Reflection can produce results in terms of learning not only more about practice but also more about oneself. Being critical can lead to the questioning of assumptions and to challenging taken-for-granted ways of thinking and working. It could therefore be argued that advanced practitioners ought to engage in critical reflection in order to refine their own practice and to lead the way in enabling others to do the same. Their capacity to do this would in turn justify their status as an advanced practitioner.

Developing reasoning skills

Fonteyn (1995) argued that clinical reasoning represented the essence of nursing practice and that it was intrinsic to all aspects of care provision. From her research, Fonteyn defined clinical reasoning as:

> the cognitive processes and strategies that nurses use to understand the significance of patient data, to identify and diagnose actual or potential patient problems, and to make clinical decisions to assist in problem resolution and to enhance the achievement of positive patient outcomes (p60).

Reasoning ability is thus necessary for seeking and making judgements about options for intervention and for making decisions about a course of action that is most likely to lead to the best possible result. Hart (1995) linked the development of effective clinical reasoning skills to opportunities for reflecting on practice. Practitioners, she suggested, must be ready, willing and able to learn using experience as the basis for understanding and for developing practice. This understanding has to come through reflection, through actively engaging the mind in reviewing learning from earlier experiences.

Practice in healthcare, as has been argued, is not a preset collection of actions that demand technical expertise without reflective thought. All practice today, most particularly for the advanced practitioner, is based on skilled reasoning and sound professional judgements drawn from knowledge and previous experience. The novice-to-expert continuum (Benner, 1984) provided a framework for understanding the way in which practitioners work, learn and refine their practice, develop their reasoning skills and progress towards a state of expertise. The rate of progress through the states of competence and proficiency to expert practitioner will be different for everyone. It does not relate to length of time qualified but to the quality of learning that takes place through reflection on practice, and to an ability to adapt and change and to work confidently 'beyond the rules'. Quality reflection leads to quality learning and this in turn leads to quality of practice.

While the process of engaging in reflection can be undertaken alone, and can generate insights into personal behaviour and practice, more benefits are to be gained from entering into dialogue and debate with others. This offers the opportunity for sharing and developing new perspectives on practice and for learning together. Hart noted particularly that opportunities needed to be created that allowed practitioners to share their experiences with peers. A workplace that becomes a learning environment for everyone should be open to such activity. Reflecting as a team with medics and other health professionals on incidents that have presented challenges can be a practical way of learning together and improving service delivery and team relationships. Practice and service delivery is not exclusively about nursing procedures. It is also about organizational arrangements, patterns of communication, inter-relationships with other environments and all processes (uni- and multiprofessional) that support patient care.

Hart (1995) saw reflective practice as an approach to practice rather than a state to be achieved. It was not something that could be switched on and off, but a feature integral to practice that needed to be developed and practised as a skill. Nurses should therefore aspire to creating a learning environment that provides opportunities for them to reflect on and share their experiences with peers and to engage in critical discussions and debate. Through these processes, practitioners could develop new insights, new knowledge and new ways of working to improve personal practice, inter-professional practice and the practice of their profession.

Recording reflections

There are statutory requirements of nurses with regard to retaining their name on the Register. The Nursing and Midwifery Council (NMC), formerly the UKCC, requires nurses to maintain records of their learning and professional development normally as a personal professional profile (UKCC, 1994). General details of how to prepare and maintain a profile are covered adequately by other authors such as Brown (1992), Hull and Redfern (1996) and Lillyman and Evans (1996), so will not be explained here. The systematic recording of experiences and new learning over time should, however, result in evidence of continuous professional development.

It has been argued that reflecting in action and reflecting on action can lead practitioners to a new level of understanding of their practice, but if these insights are not recorded then they may be lost. Much of the learning that occurs in everyday practice tends either to go unnoticed or to be passed off as unimportant or insignificant, and minimal thought is given to noting it down. Diaries, logs, journals and portfolios can all provide a medium for recording insights into nursing practice that have emerged in the course of everyday work. Novel or unusual incidents, critical incidents, incidents that have required special thought and attention, and situations that have not been encountered before are likely to be the ones from which new insights emerge. These are the experiences that demand more intensive thought and that require the exploration of current knowledge and the evaluation of previous experience to ascertain whether anything from earlier experiences can be drawn on to assist with dealing with the situation.

Developing a portfolio

Although profiles are a requirement, a portfolio is now commonly the place to collect and present evidence of continuing competence and professional development (Alsop, 2000). The word is derived from the Latin portare, meaning 'to carry', and folium, meaning 'a leaf' (Alsop, 1995), but is now more commonly associated with a collection of papers or artefacts and has wide application in education and learning (Brown and Knight, 1994). Calman (1998) suggested that a portfolio is a personal professional development tool aimed at encouraging reflection and self-direction in identifying learning needs. Redman (1994) observed that a portfolio should be concerned with evidence of good practice. A portfolio should indicate that a practitioner is using up-to-date interventions for which there is evidence of effectiveness (Alsop, 2000). Redman (1994, p42) reinforced the fact that a portfolio is a record of evidence, claiming that a portfolio 'was not just an historical record of achievement nor a current profile of competence but a living, growing, collection of evidence that mirrors the growth of its owner, including his or her hopes and plans for the future'. A portfolio is therefore dynamic in nature, constantly changing to reflect new experiences and learning. Brown (1992) captured the essence of this in her definition of portfolio which, she contended, is:

> a collection of evidence which demonstrates the continuing acquisition of skills, knowledge, attitudes, understanding and achievement. It is both retrospective and prospective as well as reflecting the current stage of development and activity (p1).

The relationship between a profile and a portfolio was also clarified by Brown. She explained that a profile is a collection of evidence that is selected from a portfolio for a particular purpose and for the attention of a particular audience. This means that whatever is recorded in a portfolio is readily available for the preparation of a profile, as and when this is needed.

Drawing on Alsop (2000, p10) the elements of a portfolio might include:

- a collection of material that provides an ongoing, living record of achievement
- evidence of acquired knowledge, skills and understanding that demonstrate good practice
- reflections of past and present activities and experiences that have resulted in and demonstrate learning
- key features of a professional career that show personal growth and professional development
- details of future plans, goals and a strategy for their attainment
- a critical account of the contents to set the work in context and demonstrate improvements over time.

Learning is the process through which most of the material for a portfolio is developed.

Exercise 1

- Go through your personal portfolio. Does it meet the characteristics that have been defined?

Skills for learning

Reflection is really a shorthand term for an integrated set of activities that will produce some learning outcomes. Reflection has to involve revisiting in one's mind what has gone on before, analysing the different elements, asking critical questions about those elements, seeking new insights into aspects of the situation – notably strengths and limitations of actions taken and their consequences – identifying the learning that has taken place as a result of the situation and clarifying any further action that needs to be taken to supplement existing knowledge. This is a cycle of learning that is underpinned by particular skills – the skills of learning – which Alsop

(2000) advocated as integral and essential to competent practice. They include:

- recognizing learning needs
- finding and using resources
- evaluating information
- observing, analysing and making judgements
- reflecting, debating, critiquing
- defining and asking questions
- expressing experience as learning outcomes
- evaluating progress and future learning needs.

Exercise 2

- Looking at your practice, identify a learning need and formulate a plan incorporating the above elements.

Reflection, therefore, is only part of the process of learning. All skills need to be refined so that competence can continue to develop effectively.

Responsibilities of the advanced practitioner

Implicit in the remit of the advanced practitioner is the capacity and commitment to help others in the profession to learn and to develop their professional skills. An understanding of the characteristics of learning and competence in the skills of reflection are therefore crucial. Practitioners should refine these skills for personal use and ensure that they support others to do the same. Some people are more naturally reflective than others but, as Hull and Redfern (1996, p98) observed, reflection is a skill that can be developed, practised and refined by anyone. Everyone, and most particularly those who aspire to becoming advanced practitioners, should view this as a personal responsibility.

Both Fitzgerald (1994) and L'Aiguille (1994) acknowledged that the process of reflection is hard work and involves commitment of both time and intellectual effort. It is not something done unintentionally or effortlessly (Fitzgerald, 1994). Reflection is far more than a thoughtful approach to nursing; it is more a way of being, a state of mind. It is not passive contemplation but an active process requiring energy to flourish (L'Aiguille, 1994). Open-mindedness to new ways of working and a willingness to learn are crucial to the process. Courage is also necessary to appreciate that past ways of working may need to be discarded in favour of new ones as new insights are gained into practice. Previous experiences must be used selectively so that improvements in practice can be made. Brookfield (1986) commented that it was crucial for professionals to engage regularly in periods of reflection, either alone or with others. Through reflection, he observed, practitioners could explore strategies for managing contextual problems and ambiguities in practice and could reflect on the changing nature of practice in its economic and political context or in relation to technological advances. This applies to nurses as well as to members of other health professions. Every practitioner must be able to modify his or her practice in the light of changes in the wider environment.

The advanced practitioner has a responsibility to ensure that others benefit from his or her expertise. Colleagues, students, team members and, above all, service users should be able to gain in some way from the learning that accrues through reflection. The advanced practitioner must act as a model to encourage reflection and learning from experience and to promote the systematic recording of new learning as it occurs.

After all, advanced practitioners are expected to be able to see both the detail of situations and the 'bigger picture', to see relationships and to make links with other practices, to be able to draw on theory in support of practice and to understand the context in which practice takes place, as well as the implications of the context for practice. These are key and major responsibilities. They culminate in the expectation that those who are advanced practitioners will be able to extract principles from situations and see their relevance for future practice.

Meeting these expectations can be realized only if nurses engage in serious reflection on practice. This means adopting habits that allow time for personal reflection, that draw others into the debate about practice, that support peer and team learning through reflective dialogue, and that produce the records of the ideas and inspirations emerging through these reflective processes.

References

Alsop A (1995) The professional portfolio – purpose, process and practice, Part 1: Portfolios and professional practice. British Journal of Occupational Therapy 58(7), 299–302.

Alsop A (2000) Continuing Professional Development: a guide for therapists. Oxford: Blackwell Science.

Batehup L (1994) Foreword. In: Palmer A, Burns S, Bulman C (eds) Reflective Practice in Nursing. Oxford: Blackwell Science.

Benner P (1984) From Novice to Expert. Reading, Mass: Addison-Wesley.

Boud D, Cohen R, Walker D (eds) (1993) Using Experience for Learning. Buckingham: The
    Society for Research into Higher Education and Open University Press.
Brookfield S (1986) Understanding and Facilitating Adult Learning. Milton Keynes: Open
    University Press.
Brookfield S (1995) Becoming a Critically Reflective Teacher. San Francisco, Calif: Jossey
    Bass.
Brown RA (1992) Portfolio Development and Profiling for Nurses. Lancaster: Quay
    Publications.
Brown S, Knight P (1994) Assessing Learners in Higher Education. London: Kogan Page.
Bulman C (1994) Exemplars of reflection: other people can do it, why not you too? In: Palmer
    A, Burns S, Bulman C (eds) Reflective Practice in Nursing. Oxford: Blackwell Science.
Calman KC (1998) A Review of Continuing Professional Development in General Practice.
    Report by the Chief Medical Officer. London: Department of Health.
Eraut M (1994) Developing Professional Knowledge and Competence. London: The Falmer
    Press.
Fitzgerald M (1994) Theories of reflection for learning. In: Palmer A, Burns S, Bulman C (eds)
    Reflective Practice in Nursing. Oxford: Blackwell Science.
Fonteyn M (1995) Clinical reasoning in nursing. In: Higgs J, Jones M (eds) Clinical Reasoning
    in the Health Professions. Oxford: Butterworth-Heinemann.
Hart G (1995) Teaching clinical reasoning skills in nursing: an environmental perspective. In:
    Higgs J, Jones M (eds) Clinical Reasoning in the Health Professions. Oxford: Butterworth-
    Heinemann.
Hull C, Redfern L (1996) Profiles and Portfolios: a guide for nurses and midwives. Basingstoke:
    Macmillan.
L'Aiguille Y (1994) Pushing back the boundaries of personal experience. In: Palmer A, Burns S,
    Bulman C (eds) Reflective Practice in Nursing. Oxford: Blackwell Science.
Lillyman S, Evans B (1996) Designing a Personal Portfolio/Profile – a workbook for healthcare
    professionals. Salisbury: Quay Books.
Palmer A (1994) Introduction. In: Palmer A, Burns S, Bulman C (eds) Reflective Practice in
    Nursing. Oxford: Blackwell Science.
Palmer A, Burns S, Bulman C (eds) (1994) Reflective Practice in Nursing. Oxford: Blackwell
    Science.
Redman W (1994) Portfolios for Development: a guide for trainers and managers. London:
    Kogan Page.
Schon D (1983) The Reflective Practitioner: how professionals think in action. New York: Basic
    Books.
Schon D (1987) Educating the Reflective Practitioner. San Francisco, Calif: Jossey Bass.
UKCC (1994) The Future of Professional Practice: the Council's standards for education and
    practice following registration. London: UKCC.

CHAPTER 13

Psychological support and counselling

DIANE PALMER and SUE BAKER

Introduction

Conversation is a skill. Some people make perfect dinner party guests, as they are capable of both leading conversation and knowing when to listen. Similarly, the nurse must have strong and effective communication skills; the giving of knowledge, sharing of information and ability to know when to listen are all essential requirements for the provision of psychological support and counselling.

This chapter aims to supply a common-sense approach to counselling, based on experience gained by the authors. The focus will be on communication skills and providing advice. Issues around the nurse as a counsellor – breaking bad news, development of interpersonal skills and behavioural therapies – will be explored. A variety of approaches, including interventional strategies to bereavement, grief and coping, will also be identified. It is the belief of the authors that when handling sensitive issues, there can be no prescriptive right or wrong approach – each situation has to be judged on an individual basis. Therefore, the most important skill the nurse involved in counselling needs to acquire is the ability to apply judgement and react accordingly.

We do not advocate that the nurse identifies the counselling role as a special nursing duty. It is a communication role, which is fundamental to any nursing responsibility. There will be times when the 'traditional counselling role' will need to be practised, for example sitting back in the chair listening to the story and encouraging reflection, supported by prompts to facilitate the flow. However, there will be many occasions when the flow of conversation will be dominated by the nurse and prompted by

185

questions from the patient or family member. The rule has to be that there will be a time for talking and advising and a time for listening, and the nurse must be sufficiently knowledgeable and confident to fulfil these requirements.

The patient with a newly diagnosed disease needs support and guidance when coming to terms with uncertainty surrounding the course of illness. Patients and their families are individuals and disease courses all vary; therefore the time it takes someone to come to terms with or face up to their illness will vary considerably.

Psychological issues

When faced with severe illness, studies have identified that people particularly at risk of developing psychosocial problems are those with a previous history of psychiatric illness. However, there are also many people with no previous history of psychiatric illness who experience psychological distress when faced with physical illness. Characteristics of people who do not cope very well are:

• those who feel that their carers are not supportive
• patients who suffer adverse effects of treatment
• patients who express continued feelings of helplessness (Maguire, 1982; Dean, 1987).

Anxiety and depression are found in up to a third of patients with a cancer diagnosis (Derogatis et al., 1983). Even following surgery, when informed that the cancer has been removed, some people are never able to free themselves of fear surrounding premature cancer-related death. Unfortunately, this fear can be exacerbated by follow-up visits to hospital (Maguire, 1995), when old psychological wounds may once again cause pain and distress.

In the absence of a confirmed rationale for the development of disease, some people in their search for answers will focus on the idea that disease occurs due to personality weaknesses, such as inability to cope with stress or anger. This may lead to self-blame and demoralization. It is possible that people who feel stigmatized by their disease may be secretive about their diagnosis, which may result in a lack of adequate and appropriate psychological support being offered.

Treatments themselves can cause problems. Fatigue is often associated with radiotherapy and chemotherapy, while steroids can cause confusional states and depression. Metabolic changes such as hypercalcaemia and hypomagnesaemia may result in reduced cognitive function, which may manifest as diminished short-term memory function and difficulty in sustaining attention.

When breaking bad news, it is useful to bear in mind that some people have a tendency towards anxiety and depression. People may offer you this information in advance: 'I've previously had a nervous breakdown', as they fear lapsing into the depression that they have previously experienced.

Fortunately, not everyone will experience the full extent of 'depression' symptoms. However, a report of mood changes, or just a general 'low feeling', should be acknowledged and discussed. Self-completed questionnaires designed to measure anxiety and depression may be useful to identify people who are specifically at risk and may require some extra support (Zigmond and Snaith, 1983).

Remember that psychological distress lowers pain threshold. Therefore it is possible that patients may intermittently experience chronic pain when there is no obvious physical reason. In this instance, patients may benefit from antidepressant medication which may raise their mood and pain threshold by acting as analgesia (Clouse, 1994).

Breaking bad news

When delivering any type of 'bad news', you should first aim to determine the coping abilities of the individual. An enquiring approach needs to be applied to ascertain how much a patient wants to know about the diagnosis, investigations and treatment procedures. A period of psychological adjustment will be required if someone is given bad news, and it may be better for some individuals to receive the information in stages, depending on their individual needs (Fallowfield et al., 1990). Many people have a strong awareness that something is wrong. However, some have no idea that their presenting symptoms indicate a serious illness. In the case of people presenting for routine surveillance they will obviously be aware of the possibility that a problem may be determined on investigation; however, if they are symptom-free, it is highly unlikely that they will have prepared themselves to receive bad news. An assessment must be made to determine the extent of information the patient is capable of receiving. Too much information to a patient with no perception of the seriousness of the situation may provoke severe distress and invoke denial of the news.

Assessment

Assessment is very important. An effective therapeutic relationship needs to develop between the patient and the nurse, with the nurse listening and responding non-judgementally as a knowledgeable adviser (Drossman, 2000). The patient should be encouraged to discuss physical and psychological aspects of his or her illness (Drossman, 1997). If patients are allowed to 'tell the story' in their own way, then contributory factors may be revealed (Lipkin et al., 1995). It is useful to allow the patient to tell his or her story of events preceding diagnosis, with open-ended questions used to generate a natural medical and social history (Lipkin et al., 1995). The use of prompts such as a head nod when the patient is speaking or an expectant look to encourage more information should support the flow of 'the story'.

We should encourage patients to be honest about side effects and not to minimize any symptoms they may have. Some patients may minimize their symptoms, as they are afraid of the implications. Therefore patients' perceptions, fears and treatment expectations should be explored. Remember to give feedback to other members of the team, particularly about psychological adaptation. Patients with inflammatory bowel disease (IBD) for example often express concern about the unpredictability of the disease, in addition to anxiety about the necessity for surgery in the future or the development of cancer (Drossman et al., 1991). Therefore it is important that all members of the multidisciplinary team practise a clear, consistent approach to 'information giving'.

When patients delay seeking information about their illness, it is often suggested that they are denying their symptoms. However, delay in acceptance of a changing situation provides time for the individual to develop adaptation and defence mechanisms (Freidenbergs et al., 1981). When patients have allowed symptoms to develop to the extent that their life is threatened or treatment is not an option, it is difficult not to ask the patient why they delayed seeking help. This, of course, is to be avoided, as the nurse may be seen as critical of the patient's judgement and actions. If a supportive role between the patient and practitioner is to develop, it is important that the patient feels understood rather than disapproved of.

Every meeting with the patient is an opportunity to monitor physical, psychological and social developments. Not only will you be assessing for psychological adjustment but also side effects of treatment and possibly a change in the manifestations of the disease. When considering the effects of a diagnosis on the patient, it is important to determine what these effects have had on the rest of the family and close friends. The ability of family and friends to adjust to the news that a loved one has an illness, which may be life threatening, could alter the relationship with the patient. Just when family support is most needed, the family themselves may feel bewildered, scared and unable to cope.

Communication

Patients need to feel in control of the situation; therefore, when information is given, time should be made available for them to ask questions. Remember that if you encourage people to ask difficult questions, then the responses may also be difficult to give.

When giving information, you should reiterate the advice given. Allow time for reflection, then go back and check the patient's understanding. At certain times it may be useful for the patient to have a companion with them who can remember what the health professional said and also prompt the patient to ask questions about anything they are unsure about. Obviously there will be occasions when the patient needs one-to-one counselling, without the presence of someone else, to ask private or personal questions.

When asked questions by the patient, don't be afraid to admit you don't know, but you will find out. Ask questions not just about health states, but also about family, work, hobbies and holidays. To be fully able to advise and support a person, the nurse must understand not just his or her interests, but also his or her culture and beliefs. It is a fundamental requirement that the patient feels that what they have to say is important to the listener, and that the listener is interested in them as a person, not just in the symptoms of their illness.

Time must be given to allow relationships and trust to be established. Time allocation is tricky to judge. To allow conversation to flow, an appointment should not be rushed. However, resources are limited and people may use your time inappropriately, therefore you may need to set some basic rules, although always with the provision of flexibility should the need arise. If necessary set a time limit – 'I can see you, but only for half an hour'. However, be prepared for the problem or leading question to be raised just as you are trying to bring the conversation to a close. If this occurs, then it may be important to continue the interaction.

For some people, the opportunity to discuss sensitive issues or psychological feelings may be more adequately dealt with in the patient's own home, on mutual or comfortable territory. Remember that it is a privilege to be invited into a person's home. However, be aware that this is an isolating environment and not always an easy place for the counsellor to maintain control. When you go through a doorway, you never know what you will be confronted with, so be prepared. It is possible that you may feel that you cannot listen any more, as you yourself feel saturated. Do not be afraid to admit this to yourself and develop a strategy for drawing conversations to a close and setting another date.

Everyone has a story to tell, so allow time to let the story be told. Facilitating techniques such as head nodding and repeating the patient's previous statements may encourage the patient to offer more data in the interview. People with IBD for example are often concerned about the uncertainty of the disease, loss of sexual functioning and fear of premature death (Drossman et al., 1991). These are all matters that should be discussed, although sometimes there are no satisfactory answers. Remember that you will not have all of the answers or the responses people want to hear. In such instances, what is important is that the patient is given the opportunity to discuss the issues, despite there not being a satisfactory solution.

When frustration is obvious, you may need to give permission to allow feelings such as anger and fear to be raised. Encourage distress to be expressed, ensuring that the patient understands that your role is to listen to their frustrations and not to pass judgement on them. It is important to establish that in caring for someone you will try to relieve symptoms. However, never give a guarantee that some degree of discomfort or suffering will not be experienced.

The novice counsellor

Using silence in an interview is a skill. The nervous counsellor may be tempted to fill a conversational gap, rather than giving time for articulation of thoughts and feelings. Equally distressing, however, can be long, inappropriate pauses in conversation. Transitional gaps in conversation have to be managed. An effective counsellor should be able to negotiate the distressed and overwhelmed patient back into the conversation sequence.

When patients drift into their own thoughts, ask them what they are thinking to prompt them back. Some patients may see silence as the counsellor holding back information, preferring not to tell them something. The patient must know that the nurse is honest, but he or she must also be encouraged to be honest with the nurse.

How does the inexperienced counsellor deal with issues such as loss of libido or direct questions such as 'When am I going to die'? or 'Is this treatment going to work?' Knowledge and experience is the key. The knowledgeable counsellor can confidently ask leading questions such as, 'When you're lying awake what is it you are thinking or worrying about?' Some people want to ask if they are going to die, but of course don't want a negative answer, so are fearful of asking the question. The councillor can help by asking the patient, 'Are you afraid you're going to die, is this what your worries are about?' Hints and tips can be gained by asking more experienced counsellors about their experiences and strategies. Practising techniques in a role-play situation will provide opportunities to develop personal style and confidence in difficult situations. As a novice counsellor, it will be difficult to remove yourself from tragedy and trauma easily; a clinical supervision system should provide some support during this period.

Teaching coping strategies

Coping involves teaching patients to adapt and manage their illness. Among gastrointestinal patients, those who view their illness with pessimism are associated with increased morbidity (Drossman et al., 1997). Discuss ways of coping and try to identify strategies that people can use to help cope with their feelings. Different personalities will utilize different coping strategies. However, remember that a small number of people find it easier to be ill rather then cope with their illness.

Problem-solving sessions or support in finding social assistance improves health for people with chronic illness (Kinash et al., 1993, Lazarus, 1993), but it must be done on an individual basis, which, depending on the patient, can require some patience.

Some people try to cope by not asking questions, as they believe that the responses may be too emotionally painful. Some ask for only a little bit of information, but then go on to request more at a later date, when they feel stronger and more able to cope. The patient may say, 'Tell me a little bit, but don't tell me it all', so do just that and wait for the patient to become 'hungry' for more information. Part of the skill of counselling is to be aware of how much information to provide at which stage. Remember to seize the moment when it occurs, as someone may have mustered up a lot of courage to ask for extra details.

Different people utilize different coping strategies. Some people may turn to alcohol or cigarettes. Some people may blame these substances for their illness and ask questions such as, 'Did I drink too much?' or 'Did I not eat the correct food?'. People frequently search for reasons as to why this illness has happened to them. However, if possible, they should be discouraged from extensive reflective periods of self-blame.

Be realistic about your expectations of yourself and others. Patients who develop illness in childhood or early life may be overindulged or their family members may 'take control' and not allow the patients to make decisions for themselves. This restricts development to the extent that they become very dependent on the family or health team members. The overall care plan should support independence rather than dependent behaviour. Encourage the patient to plan diversional activities, remembering that it takes time to learn to live with a disease. Routine plans should include how to cope with sudden symptoms. Symptoms such as those experienced by patients with IBD need to be incorporated into life's daily plan (Katz, 1999).

The patient–practitioner relationship

When providing information and education, it is useful to first elicit the patient's understanding about the disease, addressing any areas of misunderstanding as necessary. Information should then be offered to the level of the patient's understanding, possibly reinforced by booklets or videos. When giving reassurance, first identify the patient's concerns, then acknowledge them, as an indication that they are valid, and address the concerns in a factual manner, avoiding any false reassurances, such as 'I know you're going to be fine'. Encourage patients to inform you immediately there is a further problem, so that prompt action can be taken, if necessary. The relationship needs to be strong enough to ensure that the patient feels sufficiently comfortable to request information from you and to share problems; therefore there must be a large proportion of trust.

People faced with severe illness require more than a listening ear; they need professional support and guidance. They often need information to put them 'back on track' or to discuss issues that have kept them awake. Some people may be tempted to take a neighbour's advice, because this person may speak in a language with which they are familiar; they may feel more comfortable with this person and find their advice easier to understand. Sometimes if people don't get the advice they need, they will look elsewhere; even if they feel comfortable with the information given, they will still seek further guidance. This is all fine – people need to be in a position where they can analyse and put the picture together from a variety of sources. It is almost like putting together the pieces of a jigsaw.

It will be tempting for the healthcare practitioner to leave the patient to make any decisions necessary for themselves. However, at times of stress and weakness, the patient may resort to being guided rather than making personal decisions. Therefore, care must be taken to ensure that when the patient has made a decision about such matters as treatment options, they have done so from a position of knowledge. Advice from a friend or neighbour may sound reasonable to the patient; however, they should be gently reminded that it is usually only the healthcare team who are aware of the 'full facts' of the individual's case. Sometimes the friend or neighbour's advice is followed simply because they speak in a language the patient understands, so the nurse must strive to ensure that she does not use jargon, which can be threatening and misunderstood.

Anxiety

As previously stated, sometimes people with a tendency to suffer from anxiety will sense the warning signs themselves and offer information, often confirming that they have suffered 'a breakdown' before. Insomnia, irritability, inability to stop worrying, impaired concentration and indecisiveness are all symptoms associated with anxiety. The symptoms can be so severe that the patient may have difficulty leaving the house or complying with treatment regimens. In cases such as these, anxiolytic medication or perhaps even a tranquillizer or antidepressant drug may help to relieve symptoms so that treatment can be pursued. However, once these symptoms are controlled, anxiety management techniques should be taught and utilized should severe symptoms recur.

Depression

Helplessness is associated with a tendency towards depression (Maguire, 1992). People who are able to adopt a self-directed lifestyle change to fight their disease, for example alteration in eating habits or yoga therapy for relaxation, may feel more in control.

Psychological adaptation to bad news can be enhanced if the patient is provided with options and choice about their future management and care (Morris and Royle, 1988). The patient should be supported through this process by analysing options utilizing a structured approach (see Chapter 10). Remember, however, that when options are available, not everyone wants to make a decision for him or herself. Patients should be encouraged to discuss why certain options are favoured over others, as it is possible their knowledge of treatment methods may be inaccurate or muddled. For a patient to be able to make an informed decision, he or she needs to be given information about treatment options, which includes details of side effects, success rates and long-term complications. Some people will not be able or inclined to get involved in the decision-making process in any depth. These patients should be informed of treatment options and advised by the healthcare team which treatment method is advocated. Obviously, this advice will be based on assessment of the physical, psychological and social status of the patient.

, Sleep impairment, loss of energy, social withdrawal, loss of appetite, constipation and feelings of worthlessness are all symptoms associated with depression. Some of these symptoms may also be associated with metabolic changes due to tumour growth and/or protein–energy malnutrition, so a careful assessment should be made. Antidepressant drugs can be prescribed to raise the patient's mood if symptoms of depression are preventing treatment from continuing. However, be aware that the patient may not readily accept that medication is the answer to his or her problems. Often patients are concerned about long-term addiction effects, which have been reported in the press and associated with the use of antidepressant medications. There is also the chance that the patient may be offended, as they think that you think they are mad, resulting in loss of faith and trust.

A variety of techniques are available to preserve and develop psychological strength; some of the more frequently utilized approaches are covered below.

Psychotherapeutic interventions

Emotional disorders can be improved by alteration to maladaptive thinking. Adjuvant psychological therapy (APT) is regarded as treatment to be used in conjunction with other 'standard medical' treatments (Tiffany et al., 1995). The focus is on teaching new coping strategies, concentrating on identification of and challenging any negative or illogical thoughts. Anxious patients are taught relaxation techniques, while positive strengths are identified in an effort to develop a positive attitude and reduce the feelings of hopelessness. In addition, open expression is encouraged – particularly of feelings that often accrue, such as anger or guilt.

Psychotherapy

Some patients may become severely withdrawn, often experiencing feelings of hopelessness (Maguire et al., 1993). This particularly occurs when the patient has been informed of the full extent of their diagnosis and they feel helpless and can determine no reason to make any effort; they just seem to 'give up'. It is tempting in this situation to offer false hope, but this will only cause the patient further distress, as they may lose their trust in you. Potentially, these patients are at high risk of depression and if a pessimistic attitude persists, they should be referred to a psychiatrist or psychotherapist.

The psychotherapeutic approach to support should begin with a referral to a therapist who is not directly involved with the medical management of the patient. The therapist may be able to tackle difficult emotions such as resentment by the use of basic techniques which focus on clarification and conflict resolution.

Behavioural interventions

Behavioural techniques can be particularly useful when utilized to break the pain–anxiety–tension cycle. Simple deep-breathing exercises can often be sufficiently effective. However, for some people, special techniques such as hypnotherapy may be required (Redd, 1989). Passive relaxation (hypnosis with imagery) and cognitive distraction techniques have been used successfully to minimize anxiety symptoms associated with hospital treatments (Burish and Lyles, 1981; Morrow and Morrell, 1982).

Group psychotherapy

Group therapy can help to decrease feelings of isolation, particularly when facilitated by skilled therapists. The group should create a non-threatening environment where coping strategies and behaviours can be explored. Patients are taught behavioural interventions and coping techniques in a group situation rather than using a one-to-one approach. This allows access to other patients with similar illnesses and diseases and should help to reduce feelings of alienation. Sometimes art or music therapy groups may provide support, while other patients may find practising yoga techniques within a group useful.

Self-help support groups

These tend to be more casual and informal than group therapy sessions, often focusing on provision of emotional support rather than behavioural interventions. Not everyone chooses to attend a support group and, of those who do, some will never go back as they don't like what they hear, while others need the group forever. Veteran attenders are useful, as they can help newly diagnosed patients by discussing their own experiences and constructive ways of coping with illness.

A study of people with cancer found that only a small percentage of patients invited chose to attend, although of those who did attend, 80 per cent found the experience helped them to relax (Plant et al., 1987). Support groups that include staff as well as patients and their families are the most effective (Plant et al., 1987), as there is a strong requirement for a facilitator to ensure conversation is safe and constructive.

Anorexia

Anorexia, recognized as lack of appetite with accompanying weight loss, may occur at any time during illness. Obviously for the gastrointestinal patient this may be due to the disease state, for example intestinal obstruction, or, as in many instances, it may be caused by psychological shock. An anxiety-provoking atmosphere or shock often brings about loss of appetite as an emotional response. Continued loss of appetite resulting in weight loss will render a person weak and depressed. Therefore, where possible, action should be taken to counteract the effects of anorexia, possibly by the use of nutrition support and/or appetite stimulants. A collaborative approach to care supported by the multiprofessional nutrition support team will help to ensure that the patient is carefully monitored and receives appropriate advice.

Rehabilitation

Physical recovery may be much quicker than psychological healing. The prime objective for many people is to get back to work as quickly as possible. However, sometimes patients find that they are back at work because their physical wound has healed, but are unable to cope with all of its associated demands and tensions. Psychological adaptation to illness can be a very slow process and should always be considered when advising people of rehabilitation time.

Some people appear to enjoy being ill, basking in tea and sympathy. However, when the flowers, tea and sympathy fade, the patient fades too. It is important to remember that a person may look better physically, but psychologically they are still suffering. Some people will never return to work, as their psychological priorities have changed. For many people, however, their prime objective is to get back to work, as it gives them a purpose.

People with good life expectancy may still require help to break away from being a cancer sufferer, therefore rehabilitation should always form part of the cancer treatment care plan (Tiffany et al., 1995). Rehabilitation is also about taking up (non-work) activities again, such as hobbies, and getting back to normal life. People who have had a long course of illness, can be offered physiotherapy to restore or improve functional ability.

It is suggested that, after discharge, there is no requirement for regular follow-up in relation to psychosocial issues. Up to 90 per cent of people who subsequently develop difficulties will contact the counsellor directly (Wilkinson et al., 1988).

Bereavement

When a person is informed that they are suffering from a severe and/or life-threatening illness, they will experience some form of bereavement, in the sense that they lose something of value (Penson, 1995). However, it is very difficult to adapt and learn to live with a situation when the outcome may not be good; the doom of illness can be a difficult feeling to shake off.

People with chronic or life-threatening illnesses often need to divulge the state of their health to their employers, and the fact that they no longer have a clean bill of health may affect their employment status. A period of bereavement and readjustment is required for a person to come to terms with this alteration in status. It may be that a person is no longer sufficiently strong (physically or mentally) to continue with his or her work, and they may need to consider alternative employment.

Family support

The stress associated with illness can bring a family together, but it can also drive a family apart, particularly if there are pre-existing problems. The patient with chronic gastrointestinal disease may feel a burden to their family members, often due to long periods of severe fatigue, when they experience lack of personal appeal and avoid intimacy.

It is often useful to identify other members of the family who may provide support, help and guidance, rather than relying on the same immediate family members who are often very tired and too immediately close to the patient to be able to be objective in the advice. Equally, people will sometimes be best advised to seek support from individuals outside the family unit, in order to protect and preserve the family relationship.

Body image

Issues surrounding body image and intimacy are common problems following surgery or a diagnosis of disease (Anderson, 1985). The subject of libido may not be an appropriate subject for a first meeting, but it should be approached later, following establishment of relationships. Therefore, it is important that a strong, trusting nurse–patient relationship is developed. Some people expect rejection from loved ones when their body image alters, while others cannot cope with the change themselves.

Following surgery, some people feel that they have been mutilated. Try to encourage a person to touch their wounds. Moisturizing lotion, for example, will help to reduce the feeling of dryness to the skin, while at the same time providing an opportunity to touch that aspect of the body. Perhaps a patient could be advised to allow their partner to soothe them by applying the lotion; this may also provide an opportunity for intimacy.

Profile of the counsellor

When people have concerns about gaps in the counsellor's knowledge, the true story may not be established. The counsellor requires a strong background knowledge in order to be able to give appropriate information, and to be capable of directing conversation and picking up on cues. There will be some painful lessons to learn and some tragic stories to hear, but the novice counsellor must remember that she will learn to deal with this aspect of the role. It can be very tiring, but requires passion and enthusiasm. This passion and energy, however, needs recharging, so allow yourself time for relaxation and rest.

Don't feel guilty if you find some people draining. Don't persecute yourself if someone is not coping very well; recognize that you have done all you can at a particular point. Another day you may be able to help more.

A sensitive personality promotes empathy and emotion. This is normal, and almost a requirement of the nurse, but protect yourself and your family. When out of work, try to be that other person, friend, daughter, wife, mother, and don't burden your support mechanisms. They will listen to your work struggles, but only for a short time before your relationship with them will be altered and could be permanently affected. It is possible for your family to feel neglected if they get less of your time, energy and concern than your patients do. Remember they need you just as much as anyone, and you may not function as well without them.

Nurses often spend more time and get closer to patients and their families than any other member of the multiprofessional team. They are therefore more likely to get over-burdened with distressing information and situations (Geux, 1994). It is difficult to determine how close or distant to remain within the patient–nurse relationship. Unfortunately, from time to time the counsellor will be emotionally hurt. People have various ways of coping with anger and bad news, and it may manifest as hatred towards the counsellor. Regular case conferences should encourage discussion and support from colleagues, which may reduce the likelihood of one individual becoming too close to a patient and jeopardizing herself (Geux, 1994). Advanced training and workshops in communication skills should help in developing strategies to reduce dependence.

Closing remarks

As mentioned at the beginning this chapter, the information given is not exhaustive and has been written merely as a guide and introduction to the subject. We would suggest that the basic rules are that the importance of communication should never be overlooked, and the more knowledge you have the more confident you will be of your advice. Sometimes this happens only with experience, so do not be afraid to ask for support yourself. Finally, remember that there will be some people whom you just will not be able to support.

References

Anderson BL (1985) Sexual functioning morbidity among cancer survivors. Cancer 55, 1835–1842.

Burish TG, Lyles JN (1981) Effectiveness of relaxation training in reducing adverse reactions to cancer chemotherapy. Journal of Behavioural Medicine 4, 65.

Clouse RE (1994) Antidepressants for functional gastrointestinal symptoms. Digestive Diseases Science 39, 2352.

Dean C (1987) Psychiatric morbidity following mastectomy: preoperative predictors and type of illness. Journal of Psychosomatic Research 31, 385–392.

Derogatis LR et al. (1983) The prevalence of psychiatric disorders among cancer patients. Journal of the American Medical Association 249, 751–757.

Drossman DA (1997) Psychosocial sound bites: exercises in the patient–doctor relationship. American Journal of Gastroenterology 92, 1418.

Drossman D (2000) Psychosocial factors in ulcerative colitis and Crohn's disease. In: Kirsner J (ed) Inflammatory Bowel Disease, 5th edn. Pennsylvania, PA: WB Saunders.

Drossman DA, Leserman J, Li Z et al. (1991) The rating form of IBD patient concerns: a new measure of health status. Psychosomatic Medicine 53, 701.

Drossman DA, Li Z, Leserman J et al (1997) Association of coping pattern and health status among female GI patients after controlling for GI disease type and abuse history: A prospective study. Gastroenterology 112, 724.

Fallowfield LJ, Hall A, Maguire GP, Baum M (1990) Psychological outcomes of different treatment policies in women with early breast cancer outside a clinical trial. British Medical Journal 301, 575–580.

Freidenbergs I, Gordon W, Hibbard M et al. (1981) Psychosocial aspects of living with cancer: a review of the literature. International Journal of Psychiatry in Medicine 11, 303–329.

Geux P (1994) An Introduction to Psycho-Oncology, 1st English (revised) edn. London: Routledge.

Katz ML (1999) A guide for patients and their families to manage the emotinal impact of inflammatory bowel disease. In: Stein SH, Rood RP (eds) Inflammatory Bowel Disease: a guide for patients and their families, 2nd edn, for the Crohn's and Colitis Foundation of America. Philadelphia, Pa: Lippincott-Raven.

Kinash RG, Fischer DG, Lukie BE et al. (1993) Coping patterns and related characteristics in patients with IBD. Rehabilitation Nursing 18, 12.

Lazarus RS (1993) Coping theory and research: past, present and future. Psychosomatic Medicine 55, 234.

Lipkin MJ, Kaplan C, Clark W et al. (1995) Teaching medical interviewing: the Lipkin Model. In: Lipkin MJ, Putnam SM, Lazare A (eds) The Medical Interview: clinical care, education and research, pp422–435. New York: Springer-Verlag.

Maguire P (1982) Psychiatric morbidity associated with mastectomy. In: Baum M, Kay R, Scheurlen H (eds) Clinical Trails in Breast Cancer. Basel: Birkhauser-Verlag.

Maguire P (1992) Improving the recognition and treatment of affective disorders in cancer patients. In: Granville-Grossman K (ed) Recent Advances in Psychiatry, vol 7, pp15–30. Edinburgh: Churchill Livingstone.

Maguire P (1995) Psychological sequelae of cancer and its treatment. In: Peckham M, Pinedo H, Veronesi U (eds) Oxford Textbook of Oncology, vol 2. New York: Oxford University Press.

Maguire P, Faulkner A, Regnard C (1993) Handling the withdrawn patient – a flow diagram. Palliative Medicine 8, 76–81.

Morris J, Royle GT (1988) Offering patients a choice of surgery for early breast cancer: a reduction in anxiety and depression in patients and their husbands. Social Science and Medicine 26, 583–585.

Morrow GR, Morrell BS (1982) Behavioural treatment for the anticipatory nausea and vomiting induced by cancer chemotherapy. New England Journal of Medicine 306, 1476.

Penson J (1995) Caring for bereaved relatives. In: Penson J, Fisher R (eds) Palliative Care for People with Cancer, 2nd edn. London: Arnold.

Plant H, Richardson J, Stubbs L, Lynch D, Ellwood J, Slevin M (1987) Evaluation of a support group for cancer patients and their families and friends. British Journal of Hospital Medicine 10, 317–320.

Redd WH (1989) Management of anticipatory nausea and vomiting. In: Holland J, Rowland J (eds) Handbook of Psycho-oncology. New York: Oxford University Press.

Tiffany R, Moynihan C, Brada M (1995) Rehabilitation of the cancer patient. In: Peckham M, Pinedo H, Veronesi U (eds) Oxford Textbook of Oncology, vol 2, New York: Oxford University Press.

Wilkinson S, Maguire P, Tait A (1988) Life after breast cancer. Nursing Times 84, 34–37.

Zigmond AS, Snaith RP (1983) The Hospital Anxiety and Depression Scale. Acta Psychiatrica Scandinavica 67, 361–370.

Further reading

Faulkner A, Maguire P (1994) Talking to Cancer Patients and their Relatives. New York: Oxford University Press.

Tschudin V (1991) Counselling Skills for Nurses, 3rd edn. London: Baillière Tindall.

CHAPTER 14

Lifelong learning

LYNDA BUCKINGHAM and DIANE PALMER

Learning

Learning is about change; learning is assessed as having occurred when there is an alteration in one of three domains. These domains are cognition, affect or behaviour, i.e. psychomotor skills. In other words, we are talking of the changes within the domains of knowledge, attitudes and skills. From the moment we are born we are learning. A defining human characteristic is the ability to constantly learn, grow and mature in order to maximize our potential. It is clear, therefore, that we are talking of a constant and dynamic change, which affects each and every one of us. Within the professional domain, the concept of lifelong learning formalizes the process of continuing professional development with the express aim of improving health and social care services for the benefit of the users of those services.

This chapter considers a variety of mechanisms to promote opportunities for lifelong learning. With knowledge and experience, a sensitive environment can evolve, developing a culture where change is encouraged and sought. The goal, therefore, is to create surroundings in which the healthcare team work together to meet a favourable, high standard of patient care. The challenges to the nurse practitioner can be wide and varied. What follows in this chapter are a range of ideas and concepts that can easily be incorporated into practice to facilitate everyday learning.

Context of lifelong learning

The speed of change in science and technology, and improvements in communication systems require all professionals to embrace change. Health and social care services are concerned with meeting the needs of people and providing reliable care within such a changing environment.

The vision of the NHS as being 'modern and dependable' means providing the following:

- At home: easier and faster advice and information for people about health, illness and the NHS, so that they are better able to care for themselves and their families.
- In the community: swift advice and treatment in local surgeries and health centres, with family doctors and community nurses working alongside other health and social care staff to provide a wide range of services on the spot.
- In hospital: prompt access to specialist services linked to local surgeries and health centres so that entry, treatment and care are seamless and quick (DoH 1997).

The driving focus of the health and social care provision is quality and, as nurses, we have a vital role in setting and promoting standards. As practitioners, we have the responsibility for developing and maintaining standards. This focus is formalized by the concept of clinical governance. If we look briefly at the hallmarks of a 'quality organization', we shall immediately realize the need for supporting a concept of lifelong learning.

A high-quality organization will ensure that:

- quality improvement processes (e.g. clinical audit) are in place and integrated with the quality programme for the organization as a whole
- leadership skills are developed at clinical team level
- evidence-based practice is in day-to-day use with the infrastructure to support it
- good practice, ideas and innovations (which have been evaluated) are systematically disseminated within and outside the organization
- clinical risk reduction programmes of a high standard are in place
- adverse events are detected and openly investigated; and the lessons promptly applied
- lessons for clinical practice are recognized at an early stage and dealt with to prevent harm to patients
- problems of poor clinical performance are recognized at an early stage and dealt with to prevent harm to patients
- all professional development programmes reflect the principles of clinical governance
- the quality of data collected to monitor clinical care is itself of a high standard (DoH, 1997).

petitive, an organization must create a culture where everyone
the importance of, and is committed to, continuous learning
90).

A second concept promoting modern care services is clinical
effectiveness (DoH, 1996); this concept begins to provide a framework for
lifelong learning. The clinical effectiveness framework involves reflecting
on actual practice and, if necessary, changing practice. As such, the
framework provides opportunities for nurses to formulate and meet
professional development objectives. Table 14.1 provides a summary of
the activities needed to support clinically effective practice.

Table 14.1   Summary of clinical effectiveness

- Selecting a particular aspect of practice to question or examine
- Finding from the literature and professional networks and other sources what is current best practice
and critically appraising the available literature and sources
- Implementing and/or learning how to provide best known practice
- Confirming that you are providing best practice on a daily basis
- Changing to make improvements if necessary

Reflecting

The ability to reflect is a core learning skill that informs all aspects of
lifelong learning and practice. It is this feature that allows one to talk of
dynamic situations, i.e. situations that constantly evolve striving for
growth, maturity and expertise. The activity of reflecting can inform and
improve life, the self, personal and professional relations, as well as being
an essential requirement for advancing clinical practice. Thus one is able
to speak of *personal* and professional development. All professional
development activities directed to clinical practice will impact and
incrementally develop the person, leading to personal and professional
maturity.

The process of reflection can assist in the development of problem-
solving skills. It provides the opportunity for the practitioner to consider
processes that frame decision-making, while encouraging critical
evaluation of actions. Reflecting in action, as advocated by Schon (1983),
supports the notion of 'on-the-spot judgements'. This often occurs when
faced with an unexpected or unfamiliar situation. It makes sense to
consider actions taken in the heat of the moment, after the fire has been
extinguished, and reflect on them in an analytical manner. This approach
is enhanced if supported by a mentor or peer group. Reflecting on action is
useful for evaluation of events and incidents, but can also be a beneficial

tool when applied to a repetitive practice, providing a framework to analyse routine work. Frequently it is the new members of staff who question why a practice is carried out in such a manner; the reflective practitioner will be in a position to analyse objectively practices and events in a simple, cost-effective and efficient manner.

The next section of the chapter aims to provide a 'toolbox' of learning opportunities.

The means of lifelong learning

Incorporating lifelong learning into an 'action as being' means having a headset that allows you to be alert to opportunities for learning, including incidental learning that occurs merely by engaging and working with people. This includes colleagues, peer groups, other professionals, and patients and their families. Significant learning is not confined to the classroom or formal programmes of study. Reading a quality broadsheet on a regular basis can provide major information on a range of issues relevant to the professional practitioner. This section will identify development options under three headings: individual learning, learning with support and learning away from the normal work environment. It is important to note that these sections are not mutually exclusive but are organized for ease of reference. All of these sections should support the development of a professional portfolio, providing evidence of commitment to learning and recognition of achievement. The consultant nurse posts will demand a portfolio of career-long education, provided by formal education and experience; what follows are pointers to direct you.

Individual learning

The diary method requires you to record daily activities over a period of ten working days or so, providing structured evidence on which to reflect. This is an exercise that comes from the time management area and is a useful learning tool in a number of situations. For example, the activities can be reviewed to confirm the way in which the practitioner spends time and approaches the job. It can also be used to identify training needs; by reviewing situations or incidents it can provide the basis for critical incident analysis; or it can clarify the demands made on the practitioner.

Reading is a cheap but valuable development option if used properly. To read for maximum effect you must be able to identify a topic, search a variety of sources on the subject and then critically analyse the considered information. Read professional journals regularly and be familiar with initiatives in nursing, from a general perspective and more specifically in your specialist area.

Clinical research may be carried out by an individual or designed as part of supported learning by a mentor, for example. This method requires individual motivation and self-discipline, in addition to knowledge and experience. Not every nurse is expected to carry out research; however, the advanced practitioner should, as a basic function, be capable of critically evaluating the research of others and considering the impact of evidence in relation to her own area of practice.

Special projects are a form of exercise leading to the achievement of a defined task within a fixed time limit. An example could involve the need to produce a report containing a recommendation on a stated problem. A project could be set which requires the practitioner to develop an understanding of a new area of work as a means of increasing knowledge. Alternatively, a project could be within the practitioner's own clinical area, but the skills required to action the project may be new or not generally utilized. A further activity to develop and enhance an individual may include representation on a committee (Marquis and Huston, 2000).

Learning with support

Coaching is a process where the practitioner is helped and supported by another to solve a problem or achieve a task or objectives more effectively and efficiently than would otherwise be the case. The coach uses discussion and guided activity as strategies to facilitate the process.

A learning contract is an agreed document specifying what is to be learnt, how this will be accomplished and within what time frame, and it identifies the criteria of evaluation. Ideally the contract is a result of negotiation between the practitioner and the mentor and should have clearly understood learning objectives, a number of activities and a description of how achievement will be evaluated. Help with contract design may be available within the organization's human resource department; alternatively your local friendly university will help.

Counselling within the work environment can be confused with coaching, or it may be associated with stages of a disciplinary process. A skilled counsellor will be able to draw from the practitioner important issues about her life or work, and the counsellor can then reflect back and summarize what has been expressed. The process of counselling is learner-centred, enabling the practitioner to solve her own problems. Counselling may be an appropriate strategy for dealing with crises or may be used in a developmental way, for example in determining career aspirations.

Critical incident analysis is a reflective process, which centres on individuals involved in a situation considering elements of the interaction that contributed to the final outcome, for example, a review of factors that may have contributed to a patient's extreme behaviour. The process would also include consideration of the feelings of the individuals involved in dealing with the situation. An outcome of the process would identify points learned and might influence the future management of similar situations.

Interest groups are for people who share a common interest and meet periodically with the intention of sharing knowledge on recent developments. Such groups can act as catalysts for research proposals, in addition to providing peer support and the sharing of ideas. It is important that such groups agree the form and direction, otherwise they can become repetitive and unproductive.

Mentoring can be viewed in a number of ways. For the purpose of lifelong learning, mentoring can be seen as a form of 'apprenticeship', where a more experienced peer acts as role model, guide, teacher, coach and confidant to a junior staff member, the protégé. The mentor does not need to be the protégé's immediate boss, but should be someone in a more senior position to the protégé, and may be located either in the protégé's own department or in a different department altogether. The mentoring process requires enthusiasm and commitment by both parties. The protégé can benefit from mentoring in some significant ways, but all effective mentoring will result in improved self-confidence on the part of the protégé. This is largely due to the interest shown to them on a one-to-one basis and because mentoring occurs over a long period of time, usually at least a year. The mentoring process can also provide learning benefits for the mentor, as well as providing job satisfaction.

Networking is a term used to describe the linking of professionals to act as a support system. Active participation in seminars and professional special interest group activities provides a forum for discussion, clarification and advice, giving you the informal opportunity to meet, chat and learn from others. Sometimes these groups are contacted to recommend individuals for working parties, which may advise government ministers, so you could eventually have the opportunity to develop healthcare strategies at a national level. Being part of a group helps to reduce fears.

A role model is usually an experienced worker who is recognized as someone who sets and maintains high professional standards. The role model allows other staff, usually less experienced workers, to observe and learn from her actions in the work situation in order to develop expertise. This can be an ideal learning situation, as long as the role model has been carefully selected and prepared. The 'models' act as facilitators and they themselves will need ongoing support from peers and/or senior practitioners. This is similar to the familiar concept of clinical supervision, which has been extensively explored in Chapter 11.

Self-development groups (action learning sets) enable the individual to work with others on self-development activities. Typically, groups consist of six to ten people who meet regularly (at weekly, fortnightly or monthly intervals for a half day over a period of six months or more). It is essential that members of the group are committed to their own self-development and agree to work together for mutual help and support and to learn with and from each other.

'Sitting with Nellie' is an informal approach to skill-based learning and occurs in the workplace. The responsibility for learning rests with the learner. They are shown the task with some explanation from 'Nellie' and then left to practise the skill alone. 'Nellie' is anyone who is familiar with the task and has either been assigned or has volunteered to help the learner. The major disadvantage is that 'Nellie' may not be a suitable instructor and there is the risk that ineffectual or worse, undesirable, practices may be perpetuated.

Learning away from the usual work environment

Job rotation enables the practitioner to develop or broaden her skill base. The purpose of job rotation may be to develop skills which will be transferable to other parts of the organization. It is suitable for a small number of staff only, and when used selectively can be an effective and economical form of learning.

Course design as learning is a strategy based on the idea that having to teach a topic is the best way to learn it. This is an appropriate approach where, for example, resource centres are being set up in clinical areas.

Secondments are temporary transfers to another department within the same or different employing agency. This approach encourages personal development and can enhance job satisfaction by offering the practitioner an opportunity to work in another environment. An appropriate secondment can provide opportunities to gain knowledge, skills and attitudes. It is also an appropriate method for fostering attitudinal change. Secondment will allow the practitioner to view her role in a wider context. All secondments should be well planned and evaluated in order to gain the maximum value from the experience.

Educational visits may seem 'old hat', but visits can provide the opportunity to gain new experiences and information. Procedures may be observed and experienced by participants who can later replicate them in their own workplace. Participants require adequate briefing, specifically in relation to objectives of the visit, and subsequent reporting or follow-up mechanisms.

Personal development plans

Practitioners should consider their individual, personal and career objectives. Many of the suggestions identified above can easily be incorporated into a personal development plan without too much cost to the employing organization. Career development should consider not just personal issues, but also those of the organization. Contractual obligations and the NMC requirements make it necessary for the practitioner to maintain clinical competencies. It is possible that there may be resistance to your further development if you have previously had an opportunity for further education. One education programme cannot possibly prepare and equip practitioners to perform all of the required functions adequately for the remainder of their career. However, as already mentioned, learning does not have to be supported by a defined programme or an institution.

Issues such as resources required and timetable for achievement should be incorporated in the formulation of personal development plans. In the first instance, it us useful to consider aims and ambitions in the short, medium and long term.

When considering areas for development, it is worth focusing on your strengths; your weaknesses will be brought along as you advance and your confidence is enhanced. Consider your strongest and preferred skills. Think of management and leadership roles that are already developed and consider the aspects where you require further support. Do not try to be too ambitious too soon, give yourself short- and medium-term goals to aid the development of your long-term goals.

It is highly probable that as specialist clinical nursing posts develop, nurse leaders will be identified. The introduction of consultant nurse posts will provide these nurses with the opportunity to influence, develop and shape the direction of nursing care. They will be role models to the profession. If you are unsure of your developmental needs (many people are), consider people you admire; perhaps you could start by asking them for advice. Maybe the people you admire have earned that particular respect by possessing qualities that are not your strongest asset; they may be able to give you guidance and direction from a personal point of view.

Consider finding a role model or a mentor. This is easier if it is someone whom you respect, admire and feel comfortable communicating with. It is important that you learn to admit your limitations and accept constructive criticism. This can be difficult and painful, but is easier when supported by a person you respect.

Changing the culture

Be aware of the increasing pace of change and the need to consider developments and alternatives in practice. Change can be difficult, but it is essential. Consider strategies to assist all major stakeholders to understand why change is necessary; help them to understand what the benefit will be for them. Encourage an evolving learning environment. Some people perceive lack of communication as lack of interest or support. If you want to be supported then so do others; ensure that there is equity in terms of learning opportunities and that everyone understands the overall aims of the organization. A 'team' will develop only with trust and open communication. Remember that to be effective you cannot work in isolation.

Time management

Consider effectiveness and efficiency. You must have an organized approach to work, supported by adequate systems that promote a smooth service without too much effort and drain on resources. Consider your daily reasonable and unreasonable activities. This requires careful analysis of your approach to work. Try to leave a space for unexpected demands. Having too much to do (quantitative overload) and continuous long working hours can be very stressful, and is a guaranteed way to promote physical illness. Improved time management is also effective to reduce workload. Consider yoga, meditation, breathing and relaxation techniques. Plan to reward yourself with weekends off, when you do not take any work home.

Stress management

Remember the limits of your responsibility. Look after yourself, and consider stress management techniques such as physical exercise, recreational and leisure activities. You need a diversion. Do not allow the job to destroy you. Stress that is not managed will make you more susceptible to burn-out (Holden, 1991).

Your patients need you, and you can function at your best only if you are sufficiently well rested. Take regular breaks from work. It is inadvisable to work long periods without a break, so stagger your holiday leave throughout the year, rather than saving it and waiting until you are too tired to enjoy the break.

Allow yourself pleasure at work and at home. There are chores to do in both environments, but these need not be painful. Your family need you, and you need them, so do not forget about them.

Different people will react in different ways to the same stressful situation or stressor. What for some people is stress leading to strain, for another person is stress leading to mild pressure. Strain is a negative response suggesting dysfunction, such as deterioration of mental or physical health. The psychophysiological responses to stress may manifest themselves as diminished cognitive function or self-defeating irrational thoughts, which can be difficult to acknowledge in yourself. The clinical supervisor or mentor may recognize these manifestations. It is important not to isolate yourself or discount the importance and impact of 'supervision' sessions.

Role ambiguity in itself can be stressful, and inter-role conflict is also associated with stress symptoms. Learning which stressful situations to avoid may be one way of dealing with stress and reducing strain.

Ensure that you plan recreational time. A yoga class may prove more beneficial to your career longevity than evening meetings. A cookery class may provide some minor stress, but it may be fun, in addition to providing nourishment for the family. Music is often advocated for patients at times of stress; however, it can be an amusing therapy for anyone – although maybe not your neighbours during trombone practice!

Clinical learning

Learning in the organizational/work setting should take place over a long period of time, with a variable pace of learning. When learning a new clinical skill, in particular, remember that repetition helps to improve memory and perception. Pauses between practice may help to absorb the material, so do not fall into the trap of concentrating on a particular task constantly without a break for reflection. Rapid advances are followed by periods of consolidation and plateaus where learning does not particularly advance; this can be frustrating but is normal. Feedback is vital –

knowledge of results allows adjustment of approaches and strategies. Therefore it is important for all clinical learning to be supervised. Further learning may be required, or perhaps adjustment of approaches to learning. This is difficult to recognize in oneself, hence the need for a competent clinical supervisor to support learning. Feedback needs to be accurate and given soon after the event, and all reinforcement should be as soon after the event as possible. There may be problems with transfer of learning from the classroom to the workplace. What may seem clear in the lecture may not be as straightforward later on, so do not be afraid to ask for help. Just because you have successfully completed a course does not render you competent, or unable to ask for assistance and guidance.

Clinical leaders

Leaders can influence the motivation, performance and satisfaction of others. When the work is stressful and frustrating, a supportive leadership style is said to be most effective, demonstrating high concern and consideration for the welfare of staff, creating a friendly, supportive environment.

Leaders need to have style adaptability, often choosing the style to fit the situation. Effective ways to approach conflict are bargaining and negotiation strategies, which are more likely to be taught on a management course than on a clinical development course, so consider carefully the curriculum of future education programmes to ensure that what is offered is what you need. Too frequently the practitioner is frustrated with the study day when nothing new is learnt. Consider broadening your subject choice for learning.

Writing/publishing

As previously mentioned, preparing a lesson can facilitate learning. Writing for publication is another effective way to enhance personal knowledge, at the same time as supporting the profession. Select a subject area with which you are very comfortable, and try to write an article that will be of general interest. When writing for publication in a weekly professional journal, the style of writing is often chatty and basic, but requires confidence and subject knowledge. Another useful introduction to the world of publication is to review books that have recently been published. Every journal has a book review editor who will be the first point of contact.

Look after yourself!

In conclusion, do not forget that you are the person responsible for managing your career. At a time of major change in organizational structures and roles, lifelong learning is a way of maintaining your employability. Moss Kanter (1989) suggests that there are essential skills needed to manage a career. These are:

- a belief in self rather than in the power of a position alone
- the ability to collaborate and become connected with new teams in various ways
- commitment to the intrinsic excitement of achievement in a particular project that can show results
- the willingness to keep learning.

The suggestions for achievement of lifelong learning, as indicated in this chapter, should support you whatever your job description and responsibilities. The information provided will equip individuals to enhance their qualities for any job, not just the one in which they are currently employed. If a change of role and responsibilities is required, then you should be able to apply your skills in other directions. It is unlikely that any of us will stay in the same job throughout our career, therefore expect and anticipate that at some stage a change of career direction may be necessary. Try to ensure you are prepared with interchangeable rather than redundant skills.

Making a difference

The tools and strategies that have been outlined in this chapter may all be utilized in the process of achieving lifelong learning. Modern professional practice requires recognition and support for continued learning (DoH, 1999). It is expected that a framework for practice development, education and research will be provided following the establishment of Partners Councils, as advocated by the Department of Health. One of the key responsibilities of the Partners Council will be to support lifelong learning and individual career pathways. Continued professional development will need to be purposeful and patient-centred, but with a focus on the needs of the clinical team. Structured career frameworks to strengthen professional leadership will be a requirement, with a key focus on provision of better outcomes for patients by improving services. The enhancement of care will be reinforced by a statutory duty towards provision of high-quality clinical services, promoted by lifelong learning. The nurse practitioner may at times feel torn between roles; however, this position is an enviable one, with a vast opportunity to influence. The majority of everyday activities will focus directly on practice, but provide an opportunity to influence others, particularly nursing peers, students and medical colleagues. There has never been a more exciting agenda for nurses and nursing. What are you waiting for?

References

DoH (1996) Clinical Effectiveness. London: The Stationery Office.

DoH (1997) The New NHS: moder, dependable. London: The Stationery Office.

DoH (1999) Making a Difference: strengthening the nursing, midwifery and health visiting contribution to health and healthcare. London: Department of Health.

Holden RJ (1991) Responsibility and autonomous nursing practice. Journal of Advanced Nursing 16(4), 398–403.

Marquis BL, Huston CJ (2000) Leadership Roles and Management Functions in Nursing: theory and application, 3rd edn. Philadelphia, Pa, Lippincott Williams and Wilkins.

Moss Kanter R (1989) When Giants Learn to Dance. London: Unwin Hyman.

Schon DA (1983) The Reflective Practitioner: how professionals think in action. New York, Basic Books.

Senge P (1990) The Fifth Discipline: the art and practice of the learning organisation. New York: Doubleday.

Index

215